APPLICATIONS OF BIOTECHNOLOGY

APPLICATIONS OF
BIOTECHNOLOGY

Robert P. Ouellette
VICE PRESIDENT, CORPORATE DEVELOPMENT,
VERSAR, INC., SPRINGFIELD, VA

Paul N. Cheremisinoff
PROFESSOR OF ENVIRONMENTAL ENGINEERING
NEW JERSEY INSTITUTE OF TECHNOLOGY, NEWARK, NJ

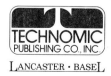

TECHNOMIC
PUBLISHING CO., INC.

LANCASTER · BASEL

Published in the Western Hemisphere by
Technomic Publishing Company, Inc.
851 New Holland Avenue
Box 3535
Lancaster, Pennsylvania 17604 U.S.A.

Distributed in the Rest of the World by
Technomic Publishing AG

Printed in the United States of America
10 9 8 7 6 5 4 3 2 1

Main entry under title:
Applications of Biotechnology

A Technomic Publishing Company book
Bibliography: p.
Includes index p. 243

Library of Congress Card No. 85-51485
ISBN No. 87762-438-0

CONTENTS

PREFACE

Biotechnology is an old science—we find examples and applications in the antiquities. Biotechnology is a new science—it is being applied in many sectors of the economy. Practical results and commercial products are developing with prospects for a bright future. Biotechnology is advancing by leaps and bounds and this new field has not yet moved to defensive research in discovery. The technological euphoria will however move from the innovative to initiative type research. In the meantime this new science will find applications subject to our complex economic and social environment. Biotechnology is currently not encumbered with a mass of facts, theories and experiences and can make its most rapid progress.

This book seeks to identify by its nature and structure both the present and future. The twelve sections attempt to give an overview on prospectives, the marketplace and selected industries and major recent developments. In addition to the text and facts, extensive reference data is included in the form of primary references and citations which should serve those readers who wish to dig deeper. We also call attention to the two recently published works in this field by Technomic Publishing Company, Inc., which were authored and edited by ourselves which are companions to this volume and readers might find equally useful:

- P. N. Cheremisinoff and R. P. Ouellette, eds. *Biotechnology: Applications and Research*. Technomic Publishing Co., Inc. (1985).
- R. P. Ouellette and P. N. Cheremisinoff. *Essentials of Biotechnology*. Technomic Publishing Co., Inc. (1985).

The authors predict biotechnology will change the shape and visage of our society. The change will be progressive but pervasive and lasting.

Few of the important changes may be readily visible since they occur far from the consumers in the raw material to finished product or service chain. This progressive infiltration and erosion of traditional methods and markets will insure acceptability of biotechnologies as perceptions and values evolve in parallel.

ROBERT P. OUELLETTE
PAUL N. CHEREMISINOFF

1

A Perspective on Biotechnology

INTRODUCTION

A man's reach should exceed his grasp. This is the story of biotechnology today. Biotechnology is an old science—we find examples in the Bible and applications in the antiquities. Biotechnology is a new science—it is being applied to every sector of the economy. Biotechnology is an effervescent science, a verdant field of research, a promise of a promise. The practical results and commercial products are few, but the ferment for a bright future is everywhere.

Professional futurologists see the future as either an endless repetition of the past or as a series of surprising discontinuities. Predicting the future is an hazardous profession, but unless targets and goals are set; we will never recognize the future when it arrives upon us. The inherent dangers in such exercises are compensated by the benefits accrued.

Biotechnology is too important to be left to the biotechnologists. Only by incorporating the view of all segments of the society, the maturing of this field can be hastened. Scientists, financiers, manufacturers and the public-at-large are all shareholders in the new technology.

The purpose of this chapter is to ponder the technological cycle; to place biotechnology within this cycle; and to predict the most promising vectors of development.

THE TECHNOLOGICAL EVOLUTION CYCLE

All technologies crawl or rush through a semi-rigid technological cycle of research, market potential assessment, financing, development, demonstration, production, marketing, and use [1]. The managing of innovation and innovators is a complex study in market and people behavior [2]. While developing this understanding, we cannot ignore social forces shaping the society and the societal trends that define much of the near future.

Five broad groups of barriers emerge, erected unconsciously within large and small companies, and united with external forces to defeat the attempts to develop and commercialize new products [2].

Technical Barriers   Pertains to the lack, or inefficient use of technology related resources, including expertise, state of the art knowledge and availability of raw material.

Organizational Barriers   Occur within the organization or firm and usually involve the communication among, or organizational structure of, the management and innovation process participants.

Government Barriers   May exist in the form of regulations, tax structure, or subsidies.

Financial Barriers   Affect the flow of capital into innovation projects that appear technically feasible.

Marketing Factors   Impact the diffusion of the new technology or the process of perceiving and acquiring new markets for technological innovation.

These obstacles are not insurmountable. Every year new products emerge from the obstacle course. Some useful lessons can be derived from studying such success stories. Some of the elements or characteristics supporting successful innovation are [1]:

- the existence of, and accessibility to, state of the art technology and technologists;
- the presence of an individual who is interested in seeing the technological innovation nurtured through the process;
- the continuous support and ongoing development of an organizational structure conducive to innovation providing the required technical, financial, and managerial resources;
- the development of government policies and regulations to stimulate (or at least not deter) innovation;
- the ability to control, budget, and evaluate the process in line with short- and long-term organizational goals.

An A. D. Little study [3] examined six research and development projects and concluded that six factors must converge for successful commercial innovations: 1) technical knowledge; 2) user needs defined; 3) existence of an advocate or champion; 4) resource availability; 5) favorable risk factors; and 6) timing of the preceding five factors.

A Rand study [4–6] reported on 15 demonstration projects in detail. Based on these 15 cases, the presence of the following attributes were related to technology diffusion success: 1) technology well in-hand; 2) federal funding ranging from 50 to 90 percent; 3) project initiative from private or local public agencies; 4) existence of strong industrial systems —manufacturers, purchasers, and market support systems; 5) inclusion of all key participants in demonstration—manufacturers, purchasers, regulators, etc.

Table 1-1 summarizes the factors which motivate the activities of individual decision groups involved in the commercialization process. It is important that the commercialization planner be aware of these motivating factors in the selection of the appropriate activity to encourage desired progress [1].

An examination of the table reveals that obtaining a favorable return on investment, that is turning a profit, is an almost universally important factor. This does not mean that the concerns of the public-at-large can be ignored. Their influence on technology deployment decisions is significant. The commercialization planner must find an appropriate way to handle the social costs incurred by a project and must find an appropriate way to factor them into the economics of the process.

TABLE 1-1. Major Factors Motivating Decision Groups.

Decision Groups	Motivating Factors
Financiers	Minimize risks Obtain favorable return on investment Compensation for service
Manufacturers	Expand market horizons profitability Maintain technical leadership in the field
Lessors	Obtain profit on investment Compensation for service
Operators	Provide reliable service Obtain favorable return on investment
Ultimate consumers	Obtain reliable service Minimize cost
Public-at-large	Social implications

Source: Modified from Ref. 1.

ANALOGUE AND HOMOLOGUE

Systems theory thrive on the principles of analogy and homology. They have been useful techniques in disciplining the mind and in organizing heterogeneous information. The practical results are few.

At least two analyses have outlined the similarities and differences between biotechnology and the semiconductor industry [7,8]. The premise is that we can learn from the successful introduction and mass dissemination of a new technology (semiconductor); and apply the lessons learned to an emerging technology (biotechnology). More differences than similarities emerge from the analyses (Tables 1-2 and 1-3).

Biotechnology is not a single science, method, technique, or activity. It is a broadly diverging family of ideas based on a few sound biological concepts. As such it is difficult to compare to any other technology or industry. It is also difficult to take its pulse and follow its evolution. A large amount of unpredictability is part of the substance and fabric of biotechnology.

The fact that biotechnology, in its many expressions, cannot be regimented, classified, and sorted into pre-existing labels should rejoice us. It speaks to the inherent richness and diversity essential to accomplishing at least some of its promises.

DIVERGENT FUTURES

Several possible future scenarios, for the development of biotechnology as an industry, can be postulated.

TABLE 1-2. Comparison Between Semiconductor and Biotechnology.

Semiconductor	Biotechnology
• Rampant innovation	• Not really a totally new technology
• Rapid succession of major break-throughs	• At the same time offering processes, products, and services
• Rapid industrial growth	• Diversity of markets
• Rapid mass production	• Variety of technological innovations
• International diffusion of the technology	• Multinational characters
• Critical availability of skilled people, venture capital, and technology	• Strong linkages between players
• Important role of government	

Source: Ref. 7.

TABLE 1-3. Comparison Between Semiconductor and Biotechnology.

Semiconductor	Biotechnology
Fundamental invention made at a major industrial laboratory	Based on fundamental biomedical research in universities
Clear military and aerospace need	Less clear link between biotechnology and national objectives
Semiconductor companies started to produce a defined product	Most biological firms are ill-equipped for large scale marketing
Substantial government funding and government first market	No such market; limited government funding

Source: Ref. 8.

The Brave New World of Biotechnology

Today's science fiction is tomorrow's reality. Biotechnology can potentially be unleashed on every sector of the economy and, over a generation, virtually change the visage of our society. A rare confluent of technological breakthroughs, accelerating economy, repeated successes, and new social values would be required for this dream to come true.

The Protectionism Cloth

An always present danger is to hide all new discoveries under the cloak of national security or industrial proprietary data. This is not, in the long run, an effective way to develop a technology. The danger of laying out findings in the open is well compensated by the synergism that occurs.

The Business as Usual Disease

Without nature and nurture, a new flower can rarely survive in an hostile environment. Biotechnology is too important to be left to the biotechnologists alone. Many actors working hand-in-hand, is the only feasible approach.

The Forces of the Market

Let the strong flower, let the weak wither, is the motto of those who believe that big business can accomplish anything. We cannot deny that this approach has been immensely successful in the past. The problem with regimented research, intimately tied to profit potential and market share is that it is a better approach for a mature technology than for a developing one.

The Benevolent Society

The central government of a number of European countries has taken biotechnology as a new mission, if not a crusade. Japan and Canada have, in the large, also adopted this model. There are advantages in rapidly achieving critical mass; there are important disadvantages in terms of possibly choking creativity given the important role associated with entrepreneurs in developing new technologies.

The Mix Model

The most likely model of the future is very much like a recipe by a great chef—a little of this, and a little of that. Different industrial sectors will behave differently depending on the perceptions of the leaders.

A SERIES OF PREDICTIONS

A series of short term predictions are presented en-vrac. Combined, they represent a bundle of development vectors covering the entire U.S. industry.

- In the medical field we will see a rapid expansion of monoclonal antibody kits. Additionally, monoclonal antibodies can be used to produce passive vaccines, to localize tumors, as targeted bifunctional cytotoxic therapeutic agents, and as purification and product concentration methods. Imagination and creativity will invent many new applications.
- DNA probes for identifying genetic diseases will be developed and incorporated into kits for the medical office or clinical laboratory use.
- A full marriage between enzymology and electronics will take place in the form of enzyme electrodes, enzyme thermistors and chemical field effect transistors.
- The ever expanding medical industrial complex raises several policy issues as to the direction of research, the quality of the product, the dissemination of information and findings. These issues will be addressed and resolved as the technology matures.
- The method to distinguish self from non-self will be fully understood and immune deficiency and auto immune diseases will be conquered.

- The concept of oncogenes will help clarify the complex problems of a family of diseases called cancer.
- Transposons and other mobile elements will be harnassed as gene shuttling vehicles in many applications.
- Rapid progress will be made in the pharmaceutical field. This is an industry with a high return on investment. While the market is relatively small for most products (some 10 million people require insulin, streptokinase could possibly be used in 50,000 cases a year) the profit margin is high, stimulating intensive research and clinical tests.
- Vaccines, targeted bifunctional antibodies, encapsulated enzymes and more will be used in medical therapy. Eventually, gene replacement therapy will be successful.
- A variety of hormone polypeptides, including the fascinating brain peptides, will be produced in large quantities by recombinant DNA techniques. The over production of metabolites from animal and plant cell cultures will permit the isolation of many promising new structures.
- On the farm, artificial insemination and sex pre-determination will become routine. Enhanced livestock growth and meat and meat product yield and quality will be achieved.
- Biotechnology is expected to help in producing a wide variety of known compounds; but most important, it can discover new techniques and agents. Diagnostic reagents, physiologically active agents, immunity suppressants, anticancer drugs, interferon, hormones, and peptides will all be produced by recombinant DNA.
- Plant improvements to develop agricultural species with higher yield and resistance to water, salt, pesticides, frost, etc., will be achieved. New plant growth regulants will be developed; and the mystery of nitrogen fixation will be unravelled and applied to a variety of commercial crops.
- Animal health care products to improve the marketability of livestock will receive early attention.
- Microbial leaching of minerals already successful in copper extraction and uranium mining will be expanded to a variety of other mineral ores if the economic situation becomes favorable.
- Amino acids and vitamins are important food additives and pharmaceuticals. The biotechnology route should reduce their production cost.
- Single cell proteins as animal feed and human food supplement based on cheap raw material or waste material will make substantial progress.
- In the chemical sectors progress will be slower and more difficult. A

well established chemistry and chemical engineering priesthood will limit the biotechnology applications.

- In the improvement of crops and utilization of plants in general, progress will be slower. A large genome, limited information at the molecular level, and the difficulty and time involved in expressing new traits will be important hurdles.
- On the market side, joint ventures, limited R&D partnerships, patents, license and marketing agreements, and equity relationships will become the norm as the industry matures.
- The entrepreneurial spirit will continue to be the essential ingredient for discoveries, breakthroughs, and applications.
- As more test cases are presented, a clarification of patent procedure, antitrust law, trade policy, and tax law will emerge both in the U.S. and on the international scene; assisting in developing long range corporate strategies.
- The pharmaceutical and biomedical sectors will remain at the avantgarde of the biotechnology movement for several years to come.
- Blood proteins (serum albumin, coagulation factor, haemophilic factor), antibiotics, neurological peptides will come under the biotechnology umbrella.
- In specialty and fine chemicals, progress will be somewhat slow because of a lack of concentrated life science knowledge in these industries. Historical and organization factors will further limit developments.
- Venture capital and R&D limited partnership will continue to be the major vehicles for funding startup and established companies. New creative methods of financing will be added to the arsenal.
- Little important prospects for offensive biological and chemical warfare are seen. The Department of Defense resembles a small country. As such, the benefits it will derive from biotechnology will cover all industrial sectors.
- Animal vaccines and other veterinary products have an easier approval cycle than similar human oriented products. The cost and time savings are providing the impetus for rapid advances. Studies are under way to develop foot and mouth disease (Genentech, USDA), rift valley fever (Molecular Genetics, Inc.), rabies (Trangene, Pasteur), blue tongue (Biotech. Gen.) and a bacterial vaccine against *Colibacillosis* (Cetus).
- Amino acid production is a vast market ($1.2 billion worldwide) dominated by the Japanese industry. Attempts are underway and should succeed to develop commercial processes for the production of lysine, aspartic acid, phenylalanine, etc.

- An emphasis on using eukaryotic cells, especially mammalian cells, will allow to produce more directly relevant metabolites, and partially handle problems associated with post translational modifications of proteins.
- Engineering for scale-up, product recovery, separation, purification, automation, etc., will be the essential component of successful biotechnology projects.
- The availability and quality of the manpower with engineering and recombinant DNA know-how will be a limiting factor until institutions of higher learning catch up with the demand.
- Small biotechnology firms will increasingly add managerial talents to the already concentrated technical know-how and will increasingly tie their research and development more intimately to the market needs. Thirty-eight percent of all biotechnology firms are pursuing pharmaceuticals, 18% are devoted to animal products, and 17% covet the food and agricultural market; indicating an early alignment with market responsiveness. Focus is an important part of marketing strategy for small biotechnology firms; 68% of the biotechnology firms are pursuing a single application, increasing their chance of survival. Biotechnology is more a process than an industry; as such, it is mandatory that relationships be established with other members of an industrial production-scale chain.
- The government is likely to play only a nominal role through fundamental research and development and inclusion of new products and devices under existing regulation umbrellas.
- In many cases, biotechnology may be a solution in search of a problem. More than 1,000 enzymes are known but a mere dozen are produced in commercial quantity. Partially purified enzymes will find many applications in the energy, environment, food, and chemicals sectors.
- Authority, culture, and style affect decision making in the industry. The societal trends more than anything shape, canalize, focus and limit our thinking. The moves toward a leisure oriented, service oriented society among many other "mega trends" affect decision mode as to product design and introduction in the marketplace. In the health care business for example, spiraling costs, and emphasis on technology and gadgetry, a more educated consumer and a desire for self help and self care; all foster the design of rapid, inexpensive monoclonal antibody diagnostic tests. The taste for meat in the American society, coupled with the energy cost of growing meat versus corn, demand techniques for increasing meat yield and quality, opening a large market for technology [9].

- Business decisions are strongly affected by the industrial sector spanned and by the size of the business. Certain sectors rely on creativity for new products while others are more sluggish toward development. No matter what, the small industry always uses a strategic focus while the large industry spent its research and development over a wide product slate. The push to buy technology at the cutting edge, the acquisition of companies with special know-how, cooperative agreements with universities, investing in small new-venture companies, and the use of technology consultants will be greatly expanded. These peculiarities are observed in the biotechnology business [10].
- When it comes to marketing strategy, biotechnology products are not so different than others. The existence of a distribution network, proper advertising and an understanding of the consumer attitudes must be taken into account. Enzymes and live organisms must be handled carefully because of innate fear in most industrialists and consumers alike [10].
- Synthetic, semi-synthetic, artificial, and biomimetic proteins, enzymes, hormones and polypeptides will captivate the imagination, an eventual rival with biocatalyst in specificity and activity at much lower cost [18].
- Many hormones exist in a prepro form. The pre segment is a signal peptide assisting the hormone to cross membranes. The pro form is essentially a zymogen and requires hydrolysis to release the active hormone. The pro form is potentially a controlled release form.
- Drug delivery systems will be made more accurate and effective by techniques such as monoclonal antibodies, specialized membranes, enzymes and new drugs design.
- The protection of the environment will remain a national priority. Chemical and oil spills cleanup, metals recovery, and aerobic and anaerobic treatment of waste will be commonplace.
- Hostile environments will be a growing source of organisms and proteins adapted for survival and activity at high temperature, low temperature, high salinity, absence of oxygen, etc.
- Serum albumin, gamma globulin, antihemolitic factor, coagulation factors, streptokinase, urokinase, tissue plasminogen activator, alpha-1-antitrypsin add up to a substantial medical therapy market.
- Human vaccines against hepatitis, A and B, malaria, herpes, and polio are being produced. Synthetic vaccines, single vaccine active against several organisms, encapsulated vaccines to sustain the immune response, passive vaccines produced by monoclonal antibodies, bacterial vaccines, parasite disease vaccines, etc., are under development. This is a fertile area likely to expand.

- Improvement in animal nutrition and product quality will be at the forefront of biotechnologists concern.
- Low volume, high priced specialty chemicals are a great potential for early biotechnology success. Eight essential out of twenty amino acids are good targets (e.g., glutamic acid, methionine, lysine, tryptophan, aspartic acid, phenylalanine).
- An expanding market is seen for enzymes in detergent, for the manufacture of high fructose corn syrup and in the milk clotting industry.
- The sale of over-the-counter vitamins (B_2, B_{12}, C, E) is growing at an annual rate of 10% in an increasingly health and nutrition concious society. These chemicals are good targets for biotechnology in spite of our limited knowledge of the molecular biology involved.
- Fats and oils important in cosmetics, food, paints, etc., will yield to modern enzymology.
- Cell culture manipulations, natural somatoclonal variation, cells fusion, chloroplast transfer, and vector mediated DNA transfer will be perfected and extensively used in practical biotechnology feats.
- Slowly, the entire energy cycle will be penetrated by biotechnologies: prospection, extraction, conversion, and utilization.
- Greater yield, resistance to diseases (e.g., toxins, pathogens) and environmental factors (e.g., drought, salinity) are of great interest. Many single gene traits will be successfully incorporated into commercial plants. Early emphasis on monogenic trait in tissue culture will bring positive results. Improvement in seed and seed proteins quantity and quality is high on the agenda; since eight grain crops basically feed the world.
- Secondary plant metabolites as agricultural chemicals, pharmaceuticals, flavoring and coloring agents, and industrial intermediates are of great economic value and will be produced by cell cultures under controlled conditions.
- Bacterial, fungal and viral insecticides will achieve some success in the field as biological pesticides.
- An enzymatic photographic process will have a chance to comptete with the traditional silver process. Enzymes, antibodies, and other products of biotechnologies will play a role in imaging devices in medicine and industry.
- Computers will play a significant role in unraveling the control system of genes. Software will be increasingly used in support of biotechnological advances. Hardware will find a niche in process control of experimental and industrial biotechnology operations.
- Enzymes immobilization will become standard in batch and continuous biotechnology processes.

- The hardware of fermentation including fluid-bed reactors, continuous flow reactors, tubular reactors, etc., will be perfected, opening new vistas for chemical and biological products production.
- The bulk commodity chemical market has been declining. This will somewhat deter but not preclude the production of large volume chemicals by the biological route from biomass and waste raw material.
- Americans have a sweet tooth. Biotechnology will play a major role in developing alternative sweeteners: high fructose corn syrup, aspartame (methyl ester of L-aspartyl L-phenylalanine), and naturally occurring sweet proteins.
- Biotechnologists will start to show the same flexibility as observed in enzymes by applying them to a wide variety of reactions under diverse environmental conditions.

CONCLUSION

Biotechnology, in many senses, is a science of shortcuts. The time between research discovery and wide scale industrial application is traditionally a long and tortuous path, on the order of 20 years [11]. The new technology operates more by leaps and bounds than by systematic plodding. Serendipity, curiosity, imagination and creativity have had their triumphs. Unfortunately, they cannot systematically sustain a society demanding a constant diet of new technology. Biotechnology has not yet moved to defensive research like the pharmaceutical new drug discovery industry. It is still in a phase of technological euphoria. Unfortunately, if history repeats itself, it will rapidly move from an innovative to an imitative type of research [11]. We can only hope that this sclerosis can be postponed until research and development has produced commercial successes.

There is logic in the current madness of poking in every corner of technology to find applications for the new science [12]. While applications are subject to a complex economic and social environment; discovery is a more random process. At a time when biotechnology is not encumbered with a mass of facts, theories and experiences, it can make its most rapid progress [13].

Biotechnology will change the shape and visage of our society. The change will be progressive but pervasive and lasting. Few of the important changes will be readily visible since they occur far from the consumers in the raw material to finished product or service chain. This progressive infiltration and erosion of traditional methods and markets will insure the acceptability of biotechnologies as perceptions and values evolve in parallel.

REFERENCES

1. Pikul, R. and B. Borko, "Summary Report: Government Impact on Commercialization—A Framework for Analysis and Preliminary Conclusions," The MITRE Corporation, Report M77-24 (April 1977).

2. Walcoff, C., R. P. Ouelette, and P. N. Cheremisinoff. *Techniques for Managing Technological Innovations.* Ann Arbor Science, Ann Arbor, MI (1983).

3. Arthur D. Little, Inc. *Federal Funding of Civilian Research and Development,* Vol. 1: Summary, prepared for the Experimental Technology Incentives Program, U.S. Department of Commerce, PB-251266 (February 1976).

4. Baer, W. S., et al., "Analysis of Federally Funded Demonstration Projects: Executive Summary," prepared for the Experimental Technology Incentive Program, U.S. Department of Commerce R-1925-DOC, The Rand Corporation (April 1976).

5. Baer, W. S., et al., "Analysis of Federally Funded Demonstration Projects: Final Report," prepared for the Experimental Technology Incentive Program, U.S. Department of Commerce, R-1925-DOC, The Rand Corporation (April 1976).

6. Baer, W. S., et al., "Analysis of Federally Funded Demonstration Projects: Supporting Case Studies," prepared for the Experimental Technology Incentive Program, U.S. Department of Commerce, R-1925-DOC, The Rand Corporation (April 1976).

7. Horwitch, M., "Changing Patterns for Corporate Strategy and Technology Management: The Rise of the Semiconductor and Biotechnology Industries," MIT Report No. 7-45-83 (1983).

8. "Biotechnology: Commercialization and International Competitiveness," Office of Technology Assessment, Draft (May 1983).

9. Morecroft, J. D., "Rationality and Structure in Behavioral Models of Business Systems," MIT Report No. 7-47-83 (1983).

10. Meyer, M. and E. B. Roberts, "New Product Strategy in Small High Technology Firms," MIT Report, 7-46-83 (1983).

11. Sarett, L. H., "Research and Invention," *Proc. Natl. Acad. Sci., 80,* 4572–4574 (1983).

12. Simon, H. A., "Discovery, Invention, and Development: Human Creative Thinking," *Proc. Natl. Acad. Sci., 80,* 4569–4571 (1983),

13. Cheremisinoff, P. N. and R. P. Ouellette, eds. *Biotechnology: Applications and Research.* Technomic Publishing Co., Inc., Lancaster, PA; Basel, Switz. (1985).

2

Biotechnology and the Marketplace

INTRODUCTION

There is no point in developing a superb product if the market is not ready to absorb it. It is essential for any firm involved today in biotechnology, or desirous to enter the field, to recognize that research and development plans and market plans go hand-in-hand and must be developed, not only in parallel, but in integrated fashions.

This chapter is patterned a little after a fictitious investment portfolio; and as such represents the personal bias and experience of the authors. The chapter makes several assumptions:

- The firm involved has the prerequisite knowledge, laboratory equipment and staff.
- Continued substantial funding is available for at least five years before substantial return on investment is expected.
- The management has the necessary dynamism to respond in real time and modify, terminate or initiate new projects based on laboratory findings.
- The company is essentially entrepreneurial and does not shy away from risk taking.
- The ability to develop and implement a coordinated and integrated business plan in parallel with the research and development plan is based on long-standing experience.

If an investment portfolio was developed for biotechnologies it would include a long list of near-term and long-term product development projects. We limit ourselves to a large-scale road map, rather than a detailed documentation, in support of specific investments.

It has been estimated that a $75 million market is required to justify a genetic engineering research program. Based on this estimate, seven market areas are seen as important candidates for biotechnology in the five-year time horizon:

- Specialty chemicals
- Medical and clinical diagnostics
- Animal health care products
- Food and agricultural products
- Energy production
- Environmental protection
- Supporting equipment and techniques

The astute reader will have noted the absence of the pharmaceutical and drug sectors. This is probably the best first market for biotechnology; but also a subject which has been reviewed ad nauseam. The dominance of large pharmaceutical firms almost precludes new entrants with the high fee required to join the club.

Our approach does not preclude the flowering of specialized companies or well established and entrenched firms in areas of antibiotics, medical therapy, or organic acids synthesis; rather it addresses less encumbered markets where rapid progress can be made and return on investment assured.

SPECIALTY CHEMICALS

The chemical industry is a 100 billion dollar business. Specialty chemicals are a misnomer, but under this heading we review amino acids, vitamins, sweeteners, enzymes, polysaccharides, fats and oil aromatic compounds.

In our well scratched crystal ball, we see the refinement of biotechnological techniques drastically changing the manufacturing steps of many established chemicals and introducing a host of new products.

Amino Acids

The amino acids market is vast—some $1.5 billion worldwide (the U.S. market is about $250 million). It is, today, largely dominated by the Japanese.

Twenty amino acids occur naturally and are the building blocks used in building all proteins in plants and animals. Ten amino acids are essential, the body does not produce enough and they must be supplied in the diet (methionine, isoleucine, leucine, phenylalanine, arginine, threonine, histidine, tryptophan and valine). In chicks and turkeys, arginine and glycine are essential; and serine will spare or replace glycine. Tryposine will spare, but not completely replace, phenylalanine; cystine will spare but not completely replace methionine; nicotinic acid will spare but not here again, fully replace tryptophan. For ruminants no specific amino acid requirements have been documented but the addition of lysine and methionine to farm livestock diet yields spectacular improvement.

Amino acids are mostly used as animal feed supplement (about 50% of the total market), food fortification (about 25% of the market), as pharmaceutical agents in intravenous infusion (about $30 million market), as intermediates in organic synthesis (e.g., aspartame) and as additives in brewing (alanine), in cosmetics (serine) and in specific therapy (glutamic acid in epilepsy, methionine as an hepatic function accelerator).

While amino acids have technical and economic value in their own rights, their economic worth is increased when they are used as starting material for higher value added chemicals. Monosodium glutamate derived from glutamic acid, aspartame synthetized from aspartic acid and phenylalanine, monobactams built upon threonine are examples.

The intended application also affects the price. Amino acids as animal feeds are worth $3–$50 a kilogram. Amino acids for intravenous infusion, while only 1% of the volume sold, are 18% of the revenue.

Vitamins

In a health and nutrition conscious society, the sale of over-the-counter vitamins has been growing at a rate of better than 10% for the last ten years.

Vitamins are the molecules of growth and health. Vitamin C (the anti-scurvy vitamin), vitamin K (the blood clotting vitamin), vitamin D (the sunshine vitamin, the anti-rickets vitamin), vitamin B_1 (the anti-beri-beri), niacin (the anti-pellagra), riboflavin (the anti-cheiolosis), vitamin B_{12} (the anti-pernicious anemia factor), vitamin A (the vision vitamin) and vitamin E are essential to life.

Unfortunately, our knowledge of vitamins molecular biology and metabolic pathways of vitamins is limited. This makes the design of a successful biotechnology program, while not impossible, more risky at least.

The availability of a near precursor might be all that is needed. This is a case of suboptimization where microorganisms might go, say 90% of the way, and the chemist could finish the job in the laboratory. For example, carotene is a precursor of vitamin A, L-sorbose and 5 ketogluconic acid can be used in the synthesis of vitamin C.

Sweeteners

Americans have a sweet tooth. We consume 130 pounds of sugar per capita per year. It is a common observation that Americans will buy anything which is cold and sweet. An obsession about health, nutrition and appearance has made Americans calorie-conscious. A great battle is being waged between sweeteners and calories.

The amount of high fructose corn syrup (HFCS) produced in the U.S. is around 3×10^6 tons commercial weight. The cost is about 7¢ for one pound. The bevarage industry uses 750,000 tons of sweetener yearly. Cereals and brewery products are the second largest user. The processing food industry comes third. By comparison, the cost of producing sucrose is about 40¢/lb. The newest entries in the sweetener market, cyclamates and saccharine, are in the $4.00 per pound range and aspartame goes for about $90.00 a pound.

A successful artificial sweetener must taste like sugar, be substantially more sweet tasting than sucrose, not add calories to the diet, not leave an aftertaste, be highly soluble in water, be stable under pH (Coca Cola has a pH of 2), and heat (many food products require sterilization) conditions, be inexpensive, and free of any toxicological taint; no product meets all requirements simultaneously.

Aspartame has been well received by the food and beverage industry. Its real competition will come from acesulfame-K, the glycoside stevioside and the proteins thaumatin and monellin.

Enzymes

The U.S. does not hold an enviable position in the industrial enzyme market. This situation will change only if enzymologists show as much flexibility as the enzymes they are using.

The worldwide industrial market for enzymes is about $300 million. The U.S. market share is about $100 million a year. Five products (proteases, amyloglucosidases, amylases, gluco-isomerase, rennin) represents practically 80% of the market.

The market is expanding at a rate of 5 to 8% per year, mostly through technological innovations extending the number of possible uses for well established enzymes and enzyme products.

Immobilization is the key word in enzyme use and is doing much to improve sales and uses. The fact that many companies involved in biotechnology must buy enzymes from their competitors, might force some realignment.

The biggest push for enzymes is in high fructose corn syrups and in ethanol for gasohol blends. The sugar to fructose market is around $7 billion per year, demanding much alpha-amylase, alpha-amylo glucosidase and glucose isomerase.

U.S. consumers spend in excess of $1 billion for synthetic organic detergents. Only 15% of all detergents contain enzymes. Enzyme content of detergents is only 0.03 to 1% by weight. The availability of alkalie resistant and stable to temperatures in the 140°F range, enzymes should change this picture. However, the difficulties associated with the introduction of a new product such as nitrilotriacetic acid (NTA) in the detergent market points out to many non-technical and non-economic factors overwhelmingly deciding on success or failure.

Enzyme electrodes, enzyme thermistors, and enzyme linked immunosorbent assay systems require very little investment. New systems are appearing daily. Chemical field effect transistors to measure enzyme, substrates and products of enzymatic reactions other than ions, will require substantial investment ($500,000 for 5 to 10 years) to resolve difficult surface chemistry problems.

The medical market for enzymes in prescribed drugs or in therapy, is small; less than one percent of prescribed drugs are proteins. The large value added compensate. It is a specialized, but expanding market.

Polysaccharides

Nowhere better than in this vast domain is the need to develop a sieve, for sorting and rank ordering potential products and applications, more apparent.

Although many polysaccharides are produced by yeasts, fungi and bacteria; only a few have been used commercially or are ready to enter the market (xanthan, dextran, pullulan, glucan, cuardlan, scleroglucan, alginates).

Three major sectors will benefit from further development in polysaccharides: the energy, chemicals and food markets. Polysaccharides are used as flocculating agents, lubricants, viscosifiers, as gelling agents in food processing, and for stabilizing liquid suspensions. They are also used in the cosmetic industry, but the most important use is in biodegradable plastics.

While addressing polysaccharides, we cannot ignore the vast store of naturally produced polymer such as cellulose, lignin and chitin.

The yearly production of chitin (polymer of N-acetyl glucosamine) is about 10^{11} tons. Chitin is an important waste material from the shellfish industry and some fungi-based fermentation processes. Chitosan (deacetylated chitin) can be cast into membranes with very high tensile strength. It is expected that the material will find application in wrapping, photographic emulsion and in chromatographic separation.

Lignin is a high-molecular-weight amorphous substance. It is not hydrolyzed by acid, and exists chiefly on the walls of the plant cells, agglutinating the cells to form strong tissue. Chemically it is a polymeric substance, basically formed by the condensation of phenylpropane $(C_6C_5-C_3H_7)$ units. Lignin is the next most common polymer after cellulose. The pulp and paper industry only generates some 22 million tons/year. A number of enzymes capable of degrading lignin have been identified. Lignin can be converted to phenols, cresols and other valuable commodities.

Cellulose is a polymer of several types of hexoses and may contain a small percentage of pentoses. The degree of polymerization of the cellulose molecule represents 3,000 to 6,000 of these sugar molecules. Upon hydrolysis, the cellulose molecule is decomposed into the corresponding hexose and pentose units. Hemicellulose is also a polymer of hexoses and pentoses, but the percentage of pentoses is significantly greater than in the case of cellulose. Cellulose can be readily converted to sugars by the hydrolytic action of cellulase enzymes from *Trichoderma reesei*.

Fats and Oils

The major structural element of lipids are aliphatic fatty acids found in fats, waxes, phospholipids, etc. Simple lipids are long alcohol chains and fatty acids connected by an ester link. Waxes and triglycerides are the two major subgroups.

Plant oils are obtained from the seeds or fruits of many plants. The commercially important animal fats are butterfat, beef tallow and lard. Soap is the better known product from tallow. Tallow oil refineries produce a wide spectrum of products. Some of the important fatty acids include stearic, palmitic, oleic, and linoleic acids.

Research and development in oilseed routes is in high gear. Microwave, infrared radiations, fluidized beds and supercritical fluids are being tested in energy efficient extraction processes.

New enzymes and biotechnologies are entering the scene. Yeasts and moulds are potential producers of fats. Some microorganisms accumulate about 40% fat by weight.

The market for fats and oils is large. As an example, the U.S. fatty amines production is now some 250 million pounds and more capacity is being added to produce the amines and their derivatives for fabric softeners, textile chemicals, chemical intermediates, petroleum additives, asphalt emulsifiers and ore flotation agents.

Aromatic Chemicals

The introduction of oxygen in organic molecules can be achieved by three groups of enzymes.

Dioxygenases incorporate both of the oxygen molecules into the substrate (S).

$$O_2 + S \xrightarrow{\text{Dioxygenase}} SO_2$$

Monooxigenases incorporate half of the oxygen into the substrate and reduce the other half to water with the aid of an electron donor (DH_2).

$$O_2 + DH_2 + S \xrightarrow{\text{Monooxygenase}} SOH + H_2O + D$$

Peroxidases reduce the oxygen molecule to hydrogen peroxide or to two water molecules.

$$O_2 + 2H^+ + 2e^- \xrightarrow{\text{Peroxidase}} H_2O_2$$

$$O_2 + 4H^+ + 4e^- \xrightarrow{\text{Peroxidase}} 2H_2O$$

Examples of the use of these enzymes might include the formation of phenol from a variety of aromatic substrates (e.g., chlorobenzene). Methane monooxygenase could be used to incorporate oxygen in methane (to methanol), ethylene (to ethylene oxide), ethane, propylene (to propylene oxide), cyclohexane, benzene, toluene, styrene, etc. Another interesting example is the well-known role of horseradish peroxidase in catalyzing the hydroxylation reaction of L-tyrosine to yield exclusively L-DOPA.

Other reactions that can be carried enzymatically include specific oxydations, demethylations, dehydrogenations, ring closure reactions, and decarboxylations.

MEDICAL AND CLINICAL DIAGNOSIS

The medical diagnostic market is projected to reach a billion dollars by 1990. At that time immunodiagnostics will represent more than half of this market.

DNA Probes

Upward of 2,000 ailments are caused by a single gene defect. Although most such diseases are quite rare (an exception is hypercholesterolemia which hits one in 500 in the U.S.), they add up to about 10% of the total number of diseases affecting us. In a number of cases the sequence of the gene involved is well-known and the mutated base pairs well identified, (e.g., β^{39}-globin in thalassaemia). It is then possible to design a DNA probe suitably labelled to hunt for such markers. This is already possible for such diseases as sickle cell anaemia, thalassaemia, and Lesch-Nyhan syndrome. A form of diarrhea-causing bacteria has been detected by a DNA probe in human samples. Possible in the very near future would be the detection of haemophilia (factor VII), coagulation factor IX, phenylketonuria, Duchenne muscular dystrophy, and Huntington's chorea. Most rewarding (technically and fiscally) would be a DNA probe to detect hypertension (the Hyp-1 gene producing an enzyme regulating the production of 18-hydroxy-deoxycorticosteroid has been identified at the Medical College of Ohio), or alcoholism (the gene for the enzyme responsible for the accumulation of acetaldehyde). The market in this area is wide open.

Monoclonal Antibodies

The technique for producing monoclonal antibodies in vivo and in vitro is well established. More than 200 MAB systems are available commercially for research and some 50 MAB kits are now on the market or are close to FDA approval.

Immunodiagnostics are now 20% of a $250 million U.S. medical diagnostic industry. The in vitro diagnosis market is estimated at $1 billion in 1990, 50% of all the diagnostic tests will be based on monoclonal antibodies.

Some of the commercially available or soon to be available MAB systems include:

Prostatic Acid Phosphatase (PAP)	Abbott Lab. Hybritech
Pregnancy test (hCG Hormone)	Monoclonal Antibodies, Inc.

T and B lymphocytes, monocytes, leukocyte	Johnson & Johnson
Viral Hepatitis	Centocor, Inc.
Pancreatic, gastric, colorectal cancers	Centocor, Inc.
Carcinoembryonic antigen (CEA)	Abbot Lab.
Plant viruses	American Type Culture Collection
Ferritin	Hybritech
Immunoglobulin E	Hybritech
Prolactin	Hybritech
Growth hormone	Hybritech
Rheumatic fever susceptibility	Rockefeller Univ.
Protein Myosin	Mass. Gen. Hosp.
Hodgkins disease	Albrecht Univ., FRG
Salmonella	Immunocell Corp.
Respiratory diseases diagnosis Pneumonia Cold Legionnaire's disease	Genetic Systems Corp.
Gonorrhea, syphilis, cytomegalovirus, varicella zoster, chlamydia, herpes	Genetic Systems Corp.
Different human blood cells	Genetic Systems Corp.
Anti-A anti-B	Celltech, Ltd.
Leukemia, breast, lung, colon, prostate cancers	Genetic Systems, Oncogen
Radioactive MAB (cancer treatment)	Johns Hopkins, Hybritech, Inc.
Fatal diarrhea in calves	Molecular Genetics
Radioactive MAB (cancer diagnosis)	Nuclear & Genetic Technology
Human T cell leukemia virus	Biotech Research Lab.
Human proteins (Ig's, etc.)	Serotex

Enzyme Linked Immunosorbent Assay (ELISA)

The idea of performing an antigen/antibody reaction where an easily detectable enzyme, (e.g., peroxidase, phosphatase) is attached to the antibody allows for easy, rapid, and accurate detection of the reaction. This is especially true if the end point reaction is measured with an enzyme electrode. I have reviewed the situation in my paper on "Enzymes I Have Known." A few interesting diagnostic tests that can be done this way would be, for instance, the detection of creatine kinase (MB form) as indication of the presence (and possibly extent of damage) of myocardial infarction. Another one would be a test of apolipoprotein A1 level and its correlation with obstructive coronary-artery disease. At least one company, IQ(Bio), Ltd., of Cambridge, UK, is building an automatic analyzer based on ELISA.

ANIMAL HEALTH CARE PRODUCTS

In the animal agriculture sector biotechnology in its many forms can be applied to nutrition, growth promotion, products yield and quality enhancement; in the prevention and control of diseases; and in the genetic improvement of the stocks.

The animal population on the farms is vast and greatly exceeds the human population. 125×10^6 cattle with value per head in excess of $200, 11×10^6 milking cows producing 115×10^9 lbs. of milk and fat per year, 55×10^6 hogs and pigs, 13×10^6 sheep and lambs, 400×100^6 chickens and 140×10^6 turkeys make up the basic inventory population. These numbers attest to the size of the market.

Vaccines

The diseases of livestock are one of the most important impediments to the expansion of meat production. The disease agents include viruses (e.g., rabies, scrapie, hog cholera, newecastle disease), bacteria (e.g., anthrax, brucellosis, mastitis), fungi (e.g., candidiasis, cryptococcosis), molds (e.g., aspergillosis, histoplasmosis), protozoa (e.g., coccidiosis, histomoniasis, trypanosomiases), cestodes (e.g., cysticerosis, gid, hydatid disease), trematodes (e.g., fascioliasis, schistosomasis), nematodes (e.g., ascariasis, hookworm disease, lungworm disease), and insect larvae (e.g., screwworm infection, ox warbles).

Each year the U.S. loses 1.5 million cattle and some 2.25 million calves to diseases. Swine production experiences a 20 percent loss and 15 percent of the poultry production is lost each year. One aspect of reducing these losses, is massive immunization. Animal vaccines are interesting commercial opportunities because of a shortened regulatory approval cycle by comparison with human vaccines and the absence of dominance by a few pharmaceutical firms. The first attempts have all been viral vaccines. Bacterial and helminthic vaccines should follow. The possibility of developing vaccines based on subunits of surface proteins simplifies the process greatly. There is obviously a large market for vaccines against rabies, distemper in pets, and against a variety of viral, bacterial and parasitic infestation in farm animals and pets, both in the

U.S. and abroad. A simple example gives an idea of the market size. Mastitis, a common udder infection, costs dairy farmers about $200 per cow every year. Multiply this by the number of dairy cows (11×10^6) and you have an idea of the market for a vaccine against mastitis.

Hormones

Because of the wide range of their actions (a recent study identifies 82 separate actions for prolactin) at physiological and pharmacological (in that sense, hormones are drugs) concentrations, hormones are most interesting in diagnosis, therapy, and in modifying metabolism and behavior in humans and animals alike.

- Most hormones, if not all, exist in a prepro form. The pre form is a signal peptide, the pro form is a zymogen. As such, they are nature's answer to time release delivery.
- Most hormones are relatively small polypeptides. They can easily be synthetized and numerous modifications (chain shortening, amino acid substitution) have given rise to a complete arsenal of more potent, more prolonged action species.
- All major pituitary hormones (the pituitary gland is the orchestra conductor for hormones) are controlled by releasing factors synthetized in the hypothalamus.
- A number of hormones act directly on DNA activating genes to produce specific proteins. This method of acting on genes has not been fully investigated.
- A great deal of homology exists for the same hormone across many species, allowing to modify a readily available hormone as a replacement for a scarce or more difficult to isolate product.
- Hormones, like drugs, cause side effects. The actions of hormones are often far ranging.
- Hormones are not only produced in vertebrates, but in multicellular and unicellular invertebrates (prokaryotes and eukaryotes). We know of glucagon in insects, ACTH in protozoa, cholecystokinin in sponges, chorionic gonadotrophin in bacteria, and insulin in *E. coli*, to mention only a few interesting sources. The possibility to clone genes in such vectors is being pursued actively.
- Many tumors produce large quantities of hormones, opening the possibility of tissue culture as a source of hormones.
- Alarmones, pheromones (under an expanded definition of hormone) have many interesting behavioral functions.

Some of the most promising areas in animal health care must include:

- Growth hormone and prolactin in milk stimulation.
- LHRH analogues as potential contraceptive agents.
- Oxytocin in the control of the oestrus cycle.
- Neuropeptides involved in pain, fear, obesity, appetite suppressant, etc.
- Growth hormone releasing factor, growth hormone, and somatostatin (antagonist of somatotropin) in animal growth regulation.
- A variety of hormones are used in preventive medicine or therapeutic actions in farm animals: cortisone, aldosterone, testosterone, estrogen, oxytocin, vasopressin, etc.

Hormones are currently used on the farm to promote growth, fatten cattle (Stilbestrol), improve fertility in both males and females, promote multiple births in sheep and beef cattle, and to synchronize oestrus.

FOOD AND AGRICULTURAL PRODUCTS

The food sector is one of the largest components of the U.S. economy. The United States is the food basket of the world. At the same time it is a very competitive sector, subject to consumers preferences and large social trends.

There are some important food and agricultural problems being tackled by biotechnology: nitrogen fixation, new crop plants, etc. These will require much time and money to achieve positive results; and in some cases must await scientific breakthroughs.

The near-term emphasis area is the application of biotechnology to monogenic traits. Resistance to diseases and environmental conditions associated with a single gene are addressable by the science of recombinant DNA today.

The other near-term practical area, is at the other end of the food chain: the food processing step. Enzymes are used in food processing for maintenance of flavor, change in properties, the removal of oxygen or bitter agents, the formation of emulsion, etc. Enzymes will find increasing uses in these tasks.

ENERGY PRODUCTION

We are a nation operating at our best under crisis. The next energy crisis will have to be upon us before industry awakes to the possibilities offered by biotechnology. Two exceptions to this rule are worth investigating; enhanced oil recovery and fuel desulphurization.

Fuel Desulphurization

It is a common observation that attractive costs at the beginning of research and development projects often soar as progress is made from laboratory tests, to prototype testing, to pilot scale operating to commercial plant. Often when the cost of a new technology dangerously approaches the cost of the traditional, technical efforts are abandoned. A further complicating factor is that often in competing technologies, the least expensive one creates a floor to the price rather than a ceiling. The desulphurization and denitrification of fuels might well be an example of these phenomena.

Of all the fuel desulfurization/denitrigenation possibilities, the microbial removal of sulfur from petroleum, especially heavy bottoms, is the most promising.

Enhanced Oil Recovery (EOR)

Present extraction techniques leave more than 50 percent of the oil in the ground. Secondary recovery is a family of techniques where water, steam, gas (CO_2), and chemicals (surfactants) are used to maintain reservoir pressure and to push oil through porous oil bearing rock to the surface. EOR is extensively practiced; its success depends on the availability of cheap meaterial to do the job. Biotechnology can produce the polysaccharides needed to change the viscosity of injected water, and the producing organisms themselves can be injected with an appropriate source of carbon and energy to do their thing underground.

An idea of the market can be developed this way: 10^4 tons of surfactants are required for each 10^6 barrels produced by tertiary recovery. On the basis of an annual 10^8 barrels of oil produced, some 10^6 tons of surfactant would be required.

This does not include the surfactants used in drilling mud estimated at 1830 tons per year; and the other chemical uses for surfactants such as emulsion, wastewater treatment, coating, thickening and corrosion inhibitors.

ENVIRONMENTAL PROTECTION

The basic protection of our environment in keeping with our desire for health maintenance and enhanced quality of life is a concern which is independent of political association, economic status and other social indicators. This does not mean that biotechnology will play a major role. Well established, low cost, reasonably effective, methods and equipment are difficult to displace until their technical and economic lives have been exhausted. The new technology must compete on stringent grounds and can actually penetrate and displace elements of this market only under a high growth scenario.

Toxic Chemicals

The simple method of finding bacterial mutants in the environment able to digest toxic chemicals to less toxic products, or CO_2 and water; is now a well established procedure. The transfer of plasmids among strains of bacteria allow to build rather useful detoxication systems. Recombinant DNA can speed up this process and give it a permanence not achieved otherwise by isolating and cloning in the appropriate vector the genes responsible for chemical modifying enzymes.

Metal Recovery

Many microorganisms have evolved techniques to protect themselves against toxic metals. The biotechnologist can make use of these evolutionary traits by selecting organisms able to concentrate, bind to organic molecules, sequestrate, or volatilize metals. The application of such techniques to metal recovery from waste and low quality ores would resolve an environmental problem while making valuable metals available to the industry.

SUPPORT EQUIPMENT AND TECHNIQUES

Biotechnology lives or dies according to the quality of the engineering associated with fermenter design and scale-up, purification and separation techniques, reagent and media quality, and the availability of transducers for monitoring and process control.

Fermenters

The hardware of biotechnology, while adequate for the job at hand, can gain greatly from refinements and new ideas. Four types of fermenters are in common use: batch, continuous stirred-tank, tubular and fluidized beds. Sizes vary from 1 m³ to 30,000 m³. A small 15-liter unit may cost as little as $10,000. A large unit with associated peripheral equipment would cost more than $1 million.

Supplies

A recent report claims a current $190 million market for biotechnology equipment and supplies. Media, carbon and energy sources, essential nutrients, must be of precise quality and exact a commensurate price.

A major concern in most microbial technologies is maintaining sterile conditions. Since most industrial applications of microbiology involve the use of pure cultures, contamination by foreign organisms can disrupt operations by halting or interfering with the reaction, or by introducing impurities into the product. Sterilizing the reaction medium is essential, and the use of steam is by far the most common method used in industry. As in other areas of biotechnology, efforts are being made to improve the efficiency of steam sterilization, including reducing the time required for sterilization and improving the efficiency through heat recovery. In addition, shorter sterilization cycles improve product yield by minimizing destruction of nutrients in the reaction medium. For these reasons, continuous steam sterilization has become standard practice in many pharmaceutical companies. Alternatives to steam sterilization (e.g., chemicals, irradiation, freezing or sonic vibration), have not been adopted by industries currently involved in biotechnology. Close examination of these alternatives may be useful now that the variety and scale of biotechnology applications are increasing.

Automation and Process Control

Although fermentation is one of the oldest industrial processes, until recently, attempts to control fermentation have remained more of an art than a science. With the advent of instruments and systems to monitor the reaction, this situation is changing, and a new generation of fermentation plants is being developed, based on the principle of process optimization through feedback control. Coupled with minicomputers, fermentation processes will eventually be controlled in a truly continuous close-loop fashion. At the present, our understanding of the dynamics of microbial growth and metabolism are not advanced enough to model reaction conditions; therefore, on-line control over the near-term will be highly dependent on the development of reliable, accurate, sensitive, and rapid sensors to obtain real-time data. Sensors for monitoring the physical environment (e.g., temperature, pressure, etc.), have been developed and are used in commercial systems to take measurements directly under sterile conditions. Sensors for the chemical and biological environment are at a much earlier state of development.

Product Concentration, Purification, Separation and Recovery

The separation and purification of products pose special problems in biotechnology:

• many bioproducts are chemically fragile
• products are usually dissolved in large quantities of water or held in cells
• in some cases, the microbial cells are the desired product
• multiple products of many bioreactions must be separated without destruction or change in activity.

Product separation costs vary according to the application, but are usually the main cost factor in any process. To address these problems and reduce the contribution of downstream processing to total cost, methods are needed that have some or all of the following characteristics:

• high product recovery
• reliability and insensitivity to variation in stream quality
• ability to process in pace with reactor operation (i.e., minimum storage or holdup)
• low cost and energy requirements; and
• capability for recycling of medium or biological catalyst.

The separation processes of industrial importance are the following:

Membrane methods
  reverse osmosis
  ultrafiltration
  microfiltration
  liquid membranes
  electrodialysis
  gas separation

Mechanical methods
  ultracentrifugation
  filtration

Liquid-gas-solid extraction methods
  absorption
  adsorption
  chromatography

solvent extraction
supercritical fluid extraction

Heat treatment methods
  distillation
  evaporation
  drying systems
  freeze crystallization

Electric/magnetic methods
  electrophoresis
  electromagnetic separation
  electrofiltration
  electro coagulation
  electrostatic separation
  electro magnetic energy dryers

CONCLUSION

Taking the pulse of the market and knowing the competition are essential elements of research and development. The sweetener market is a good example. A glut of sucrose exists today with depressed prices. The development of noncaloric sweeteners will further depress the market. Is it then time to look into a sucrochemistry to replace high valued added petroleum derived products? Some 10,000 derivatives of sucrose are known. Some 100 products appear to have industrial value. A mere dozen have faired well in the market.

Another example is the production of essential amino acids as food additive competing with attempts to incorporate genes for such amino acids in new corn and soybean plants.

System analysis should come to the rescue of the harassed businessman and curious and imaginative scientist in helping, in a structured and disciplined fashion, to select and stabilize targets of opportunity for biotechnology.

Among the criteria to be considered, the following must play a prominent role:

The Market

- Its size
- Its dominance by a few giants or not
- Its level of "captivity" in hard-wired relationships between firms
- Its growth rate
- Its stability or variability or seasonability
- The share expected to be captured by the new products
- Replacement, substitution market or new market

The Risk

- Level of technical difficulties—are breakthroughs required?
- Requirement for new technology or method
- New skills or manpower required

The Timing

- Time to commercial success
- Return on investment period
- Is this timing in synch with the growth, retooling, expansion cycle of the relevant industry?

The Costs

* Total investment required
* Current sunken costs
* R&D cost as a ratio of future sales

The failure of success is not a problem yet for biotechnology. Some $2 billion of research and development funds are being poured into biotechnology. How judiciously are the moneys used, will define the future.

3

The Diseases of Biotechnology

The patient is showing unusual symptoms. Born, from a large-scale industrial point of view, only a few years ago, biotechnology is already sick. The symptomatology is worth describing; the diagnosis might lead to timely therapy.

The patient is in guarded condition. Upon close scrutiny, new symptoms are discovered. While the prognosis is good, a long and complex treatment course must be prescribed and recovery must be closely monitored to avoid relapse.

THE *E. COLI* SYNDROME

Bacteria are phenomenal factories. With a surface to volume ratio of the order of 100,000 (it is roughly 0.3 for a man); a metabolism allowing them to consume 10,000 times their weight in lactose per hour (a man would require 250 hours to consume its own weight in sugar); a rapid sexual multiplication rate, doubling every 20 minutes (a human generation is some 25 years); and an inexpensive diet of carbon and nitrogen; they are made to order.

Biologists have been studying the common bacteria *Escherichia coli* with an almost vengeful, relentless determination. After man, it is the best studied organism. A vast bank of knowledge has been accumulated on this workhorse of biotechnology as to growth conditions, plasmid sequences, membrane structure and gene expression. Unfortunately, as ideal as *E. coli* is for biological studies, it is a poor engineering solution.

Our favorite bacteria is a potential pathogenic agent as a normal inhabitant of the human digestive tract. It does not export or secrete proteins into its environment (by comparison, *Bacillus subtilis* can secrete over 50 different antibiotics). It contains highly toxic endotoxins. It operates in a narrow range of environmental conditions (temperature, pH, salinity, etc.). It can be grown in culture only in limited density. Interesting mutants often revert to wild types. Other organisms are more tolerant or thrive under adverse conditions.

While some of the above problems have been overcome in *E. coli* research, *E. coli* is not the ideal factory for routine industrial operations.

What are the alternative organisms? There are four broad classes of industrially interesting micro-organisms; molds, yeasts, single cell bacteria and actinomycetes. More than 100,000 species of micro-organisms exist in nature. Their metabolic pathways are diverse. We should make use of the diversity provided by nature. Xanthan is synthesized by the bacterium *Xanthomonas campesta*; the acetone-butanol fermentation is catalyzed by the bacterium *Clostridium acetobutylicum*; the enzyme glucomylase is extracted from *Aspergillus niger*; penicillin is produced from the mold *Penicillium chrysogenum*; riboflavin is overproduced by the mold *Ashbya gussypii*; rennin is mostly extracted from *Mucor pusilus*; and lysine is obtained from *Corynebacterium glutamicum*.

Some microorganisms perform interesting and potentially valuable functions. The fungi ascomycete *Chaetomium* can digest cellulose, strains of the "superbug" *Pseudomonas putida* thrive on petroleum, and members of the *Thiobacillus* generally can assist in mineral leaching operations.

Many molecules of interest, such as alkaloids, plant growth factors, and toxins, are produced by one or a few lesser known and yet industrially well behaved organisms. We have to learn to use such organisms.

Microorganisms are being induced to produce chemicals that nature never produced, thus filling the void between the availability of natural products and the increasing difficulty to *de novo* synthesize large and potentially complex new chemicals.

All organisms can be "taught" to overproduce large quantities of a desired product by acting on their environment or their genetic make-up (e.g., by tinkering with their operon control system or by amplification of the specific plasmid).

Increasingly, new microorganisms besides *E. coli* are being used as hosts for foreign DNA: the free living soil species of *Azotobacter, Rhizobium* living symbiotically on roots and the spore forming strict aerobic bacteria *Bacillus subtilis* have all been used successfully.

Nature is an immense laboratory never rivaled by man's feeble attempts. If we travel into this laboratory we find microorganisms living under the most varied conditions from the freezing point to near the boiling point of water; in fresh and in salt water; with or without oxygen. Our environment provides a broad range of ecological niches. Within that limit, nature as engineer provides diversity by variation on a few favorite themes.

Highly engineered cells bear little resemblence to their ancestors. The bacteria as the hosts of the future will be improvements on nature combining the most useful traits, characteristics, and properties from nature's menu.

THE WATER SYNDROME

A biologist is a person obsessed with water. He operates in an aqueous environment, isotonic, buffered and in a narrow range of temperature and pressure.

This historical orientation, more than an actual requirement, makes the difficult step of purification the more difficult and costly since large volumes of liquid must be treated to extract a small amount of usable product.

Indeed many proteins, primary and secondary metabolites are soluble in water and observed reactions in biological systems are in an aqueous phase.

Immobilization of enzymes and cells through adsorption on surfaces, entrapment in polymeric gel, copolymerization or cross-linking with bifunctional reagents, covalent attachment to solid support and encapsulation, will help move the organisms and their active agents from a dilute to a more concentrated environment. The net result of immobilization is to convert enzymes from a water soluble to a water insoluble status. Additional advantages are secured such as reuse of the enzyme and easy utilization of conventional chemical reactors.

Additionally, cells and enzymes are removed from an often hostile environment and are afforded additional protection against the action of proteases, autolysis, mechanical stress, pH denaturation, oxygen scavenging, thermal inactivation and modification in their stability (too often in the wrong direction). Immobilization provides a microenvironment that can be substantially different in terms of charge, ionic strength, pH, etc., than the bulk phase.

Enzymes are useful molecules because of their specific activity and stability. Otherwise they are mundane. Stability is the cornerstone of the edifice. Stability has many meanings: thermostability, heat lability and temperature optimum; pH range and optimum; resistance to destruction by proteolytic enzymes; the need for (adenosine triphosphate and nicotinamide-derived species) cofactors, the reaction rate; the role of water and other solvents; inhibition (competitive, non-competitive, mixed) by substrate analog molecules or by reaction products. Each facet of stability must be taken into account in engineering an enzyme system. This is especially true, the further we move away from physiological conditions.

It has been repeatedly demonstrated that some enzymes can function properly at liquid-liquid interfaces or in the presence of organic solvents. Studies have shown that the reaction mechanisms established in more physiological conditions, that is in aqueous solution, were not modified by the presence of organic solvents including antifreeze. Murine fibroblast cell lines and human newborn foreskin fibroblasts have been grown at the interface between water and hydrophobic fluids such as fluorocarbon and silicone fluids. They have been found to be well suited to provide cell growth on an inert, non-toxic, hydrophobic substrate.

Further, many of the molecules of interest, e.g., steroids, are not or are only partially miscible with water. As usual, biology presents us with a range of problems and a spectrum of solutions.

Liquids are known to exhibit extreme selectivities between chemically related species. The recognition of this basic fact has led investigators to design liquid membranes (support-type and emulsion type) to take full advantage of the broad range of properties.

These membranes have tremendous potential for biotechnology. Liquid membranes are capable of moving a solute from a region of high concentration into a region of low concentration. They can separate two miscible liquids and can control the mass transfer between these liquids. The membrane provides a large interfacial area. They provide a kind of extraction phenomenon in which the solute capacity of a dispersed solvent is increased by the addition of islands of an irreversibly reactive material. They obviously can also be used for enzyme immobilization and time release of chemicals.

We have open to us a variety of compromises along a spectrum from dilute aqueous to concentrated aqueous solutions and from water based to organic based media.

Enzymes are sometimes stored in organic solvent to protect them from degradation. It is only a step, though a giant one, to teach enzymes to become operational in the absence of water.

THE ENGINEERING SYNDROME

Science is outpacing engineering and the gap is becoming larger with passing years. Some of the major engineering challenges facing biotechnology include the pretreatment of feedstock, the design of large scale fermenters, the installation of continuous systems, the direct and indirect measurement of properties of the reactions under way, the gentle but efficient product separation, purification and recovery, and the automation of the factory.

The most difficult and the most tedious problems of molecular biology is dealing with separation, purification, concentration, isolation. High efficiency, fast, repeatable and gentle methods are needed.

Optimization of growth conditions for microorganisms and optimization of the process and equipment will be required to realize the promised gains in material, energy and cost savings.

The possibility of completing chemical reactions under gentler conditions might have obscured the well-known fact that temperature enhances reaction rates. A compromise is being sought by searching for and selecting organisms which operate at higher temperature and under a wider range of pH conditions. Thermophilic organisms such as *Clostridium thermocellum* thrive at 55–60 °C in the absence of oxygen, simultaneously hydrolyzing cellulose to glucose and fermenting it to ethanol. *Thermoanaerobacter ethanolicus*, collected from natural hot springs, converts glucose to ethanol at 78 °C versus the traditional operation at 37 °C. The reverse side is that enzymes from organisms acclimated to low temperatures have smaller activation energy and greater activity.

A well-known principle in engineering is that costs increase exponentially from concept, to systems study, to laboratory model, to pilot plant, to production facility. If scale-up laws were linear and well behaved, engineering would be no fun at all. Engineers are indeed happy with many years of problems to solve. This holds true for engineering/biology as well.

The merging of solid state electronics and bioprocessing may hold the key to solving many of the engineering problems mentioned. Toward this end, the combination of selective membranes and enzymes with field effect transistors has given rise to a new species, the ChemFET— The Chemical Field Effect Transistor. This device combines the chemical specificity of immobilized enzymes with the ability of semiconductor transistors to sense small changes in electric potential associated with ion movements, pH changes or other electrochemical phenomena. Discoveries more often than not occur at the interface between particular sciences. The IsFET and ChemFET are encouraging examples.

Engineering has solved many problems of sterilization by chemical treatment; separation and concentration by membranes, (ultrafiltration, reverse osmosis, liquid/liquid membranes), by supercritical

CO_2, by affinity chromatography; and measurement of process parameters by chemical field effect transistors; to mention only a few solutions in search of problems.

Engineering lacks the glamour of experimental research. Biotechnology will live or die not in the test tubes of the biochemists but on the workbench of the biochemical engineers. Engineers have faced such challenges before with great success in chemistry, limited progress in medicine, and dismal failure in tackling social problems such as crime and population control.

The need to develop a common language between engineers and biologists, to erect permanent bridges between the disciplines, and to work at the interfaces between the sciences has never been so great. When and how this is achieved will spell success or failure.

THE ENTHUSIASM SYNDROME

The enthusiasts, in any field, are its best friends and its worst enemies. They light the fire, carry the torch, rekindle the interest and blow gently on cooling ashes. But they also foster, by exaggerated claims, an accumulation of disappointments in the general public, frustrations in investigators, and a shying away of prudent investors. A return to reality is imperative.

There is a rule of thumb in estimating the time needed to develop complex software. You ask your three best systems analysts for a time estimate. You discard the lowest two and multiply the last one by the square root of three. The same applies to biotechnology. All that has been suggested can be developed; but the lead time will be much longer than currently estimated.

It is easy to become excited at news of a super mouse containing an injected growth hormone gene, the development of a human blood replacement, the design of a contraceptive vaccine, the availability of monoclonal antibody kits to detect sexually transmitted pathogens: *Neisseria gonorrhoeae* (gonorrhoea), *Chlamydia trachomatis* (pelvic infection disease) and *Herpesviridae* (herpes simplex virus infection), the testing of mass produced interferon, the marketing of Humulin (insulin produced by recombinant DNA techniques), and the goal of crispier french fries and juicier tomatoes.

All these items and more have appeared in recent months in technical articles in reputed scientific publications; to be echoed in such journals as the *Wall Street Journal* and the *New York Times* and such magazines as *Science Digest* and *Science 83*.

The scientific community and the public are exposed to a barrage of ideas, concepts and realizations firing the imagination. Enthusiasm is a communicative disease. It is as essential to the scientist as instruments and methods. But, enthusiasm must be tempered with realism.

THE BUG SYNDROME

In the struggle for existence, more often than not, the plants lose to the animals. In the biotechnology game the higher plants have been losing ground to bacteria, fungi and yeast.

A plant is so much more complex than a bacterium. Progress has been slower but gains are reported daily.

Propagation of plant organs, tissues and cells in culture has been achieved. Clonal multiplication of plants, protoplast fusion and the introduction of foreign DNA have all been achieved. Somatic cell fusion techniques permits the genome of sexually incompatible species to be united. Somatic hybrid plants from fusions have given rise to promising "topatoes" and "pomatoes." Individual genes have been transferred between prokaryotes and eukaryotes. These techniques are routine in only a few species, however.

Increased yield, nutritional quality of grains, disease and toxin resistance, past resistance, tolerance to herbicides, decreased photorespiration, drought and salt resistance, timing of flowering and maturity are traits of great economic interests.

Many traits of agronomic importance are the product of organization and differentiation of cells and can be expressed only in the mature organisms.

Genetic manipulation is useuless unless the new trait can be expressed in the mature plant. Here lies a new layer of difficulty.

THE MARKET SYNDROME

Estimates of the potential market are growing with each new expert estimate provided. How come so few people are making real money?

Most commentators agree that biotechnological development in the next decade will be deominated by high value added products in fine chemicals and pharmaceuticals.

To take money in the biotechnology field you will need money, luck and patience. In most cases, substantial R&D needs, untested engineering and production concepts, competition with established products, and an ill-defined government regulatory process face the new company and its financial backers.

A few biotechnology companies are offering stocks. After a rush for such glamorous offering, reality has set in and the stock values have fallen to more reasonable levels.

A variety of innovative financing techniques such as R&D limited partnerships are being tested by young biotechnology companies. Venture capital has been attracted by such propositions.

Money is the great common denominator and equalizer. Biotechnology will soar only if investors are patient and if early profits are realized and reinvested into research, demonstration and development.

The needed funds to develop the engineering will be the largest. This is the acid test of biotechnology. This is the frontier.

THE UNIVERISTY-INDUSTRY SYNDROME

In the good old days university professors never spoke to industrialists and as rarely as possible to their students. Their interest was pure research. Industrialists heap scorn on the poor absentminded, impractical intellectuals. The world was simple. These barriers have been broken down. The university is in danger of becoming a mere stepping stone to higher wages and ownership in the industry with attendant losses in fundamental science.

The debate is intensifying over conflicts of interest at major university research centers. Most universities have conflict of interest policies concerning financial relationship of professors to corporations that also sponsor their research. The fear is that corporations might slow university research or limit the publication of technical findings with eventual commercial value. Spokesmen from academia have emphasized three guiding principles: academic freedom, university autonomy in academic affairs and institutional neutrality. The salient point has been made that with government sponsored research, academic institutions have readily accepted government policies without having to resolve the conflict of interest issue; since the government can be presumed to represent the public interest. In the case of industrial funding, the institutions must accept the responsibility of directly dealing with conflict avoidance and resolution.

On the other side of the coin, numerous universities are signing cooperative agreements with commercial firms joining efforts in new science advancement and products development. This is a desirable state of affairs.

The balance between the need for alternative research funds from the industry to offset reductions in government funding and the sacred academic freedom will not be resolved easily.

Problems of science cannot be solved by politics; but the politics of science cannot be ignored. Nowhere is this more evident than in government funding of research. Established scientists laboring in safe areas of research capture the largest piece of the pie, leaving the younger, lesser known investigators to play a secondary role in discovery. The trend must be reversed if we are to continue reaping benefits from research.

THE WASTE AS A RAW MATERIAL SYNDROME

A number of scientists have tackled the conversion of waste material into useful products. Alcohols, high fructose syrup, and single cell proteins are only a few dramatic examples.

The premise is that we can solve an environmental problem and at the same time have access to an inexpensive, plentiful source of raw material.

A waste is a resource out of place. Wastes, like products, respond to the basic economics law of supply and demand. As soon as a waste is demanded, the price will climb and the economic balance sheet of many new processes is likely to suffer. In addition, it is not unusual in a biomass to alcohol conversion program to find out that the acquisition, collection, and transportation of the waste material is the dominant factor in operation costs.

THE EDUCATED INCAPACITY SYNDROME

This beautiful statement from Herman Kahn is fully applicable to biotechnology. Many biotechnology companies are competing in recruiting able scientists, technicians and managers. Curricula in biotechnology are inadequate. Experimentally trained and theroetically well grounded teachers do not exist. Students are rarely receiving proper guidance from their counsellors.

In the normal industrial evolution, a point is reached where skill is more in demand than knowledge. Biotechnology is evolving at such a rapid pace that we are in danger of foregoing the fundamentals (e.g., biochemistry, enzymology) for applied studies (e.g., genetic engineering).

Who will train the new generation of scientists and technologists? Who will teach them to think "non-linearly," to depart from established paths, to violate dogma? The universities are slowly awakening to their responsibilities.

THE SCIENTIFIC SNOBBERY SYNDROME

Science has replaced religion in shaping society. Scientists have received increasing powers with attendant responsibilities.

Scientists are too often insensitive to laymen concerns discounting them as irrational. This scientific snobbery has given rise to accusations of playing God with the stuff of life.

Genetic engineering is not only seen as a danger to life, it is perceived as an assault on cherished traditional values. It is for many an unwanted knowledge.

A myriad of social and ethical issues arise out of the unpredictability of the new technology. The speed of evolution of the new knowledge is the most disturbing to the uninitiated. A gargantuan effort in the public press must be made to educate the public without passion and exaggeration so common to such reporting.

The issue of risk cannot be ignored as gene splicing is employed in manufacturing, agriculture, medical treatment and is introduced accidentally and willfully in the general environment. We lack the infrastructure to deal with such potential problems or catastrophes.

Specialists are accepted as a necessity but are rarely trusted by the public. Scientists cannot afford to be smug about hazards—we know so little. Even if some public concerns are not supported by scientific evidence, they have to be addressed somehow. Remember that insensitivity from the scientific community virtually killed the nuclear industry in this country. It would be a shame to have learned so little from recent history.

The way biotechnology is perceived (and we live in a world of perceptions) by the public will affect and even define the response of the market place, the availability of funds and the intensity of government regulations.

Scientists must anticipate and blunt potential confrontation and diffuse acrimonious debate by a systematic review of risk and hazards and by the erection of protective barriers. Future problems cannot be left to future generations but must be tackled now with our imperfect knowledge and tools.

A PERSPECTIVE

What is the prognosis for our patient? Knowing the size and dimension of a problem is one-half of the solution. We have attempted to characterize the difficulties and have outlined possible therapeutic actions. The patient will live and prosper if all the practitioners apply their knowledge, skill and devotion.

A ferment is spreading over the land; new ideas are brewing; this is the age of industrial microbiology.

The world has experienced many revolutions, many waves, many changes. It is probably the better for them. The invention of the wheel, the engineering of the automobile, the advent of space travel and the miniaturization of electronics are landmarks in the exploding social evolution. Is biotechnology the next societal change? Is it similar to the previous examples? Is it different from them in degree or kind of impact? Only time will tell. If we have learned one thing during our tortuous evolution it is that we can manage and shape the future.

Biotechnology as a phenomenum is as old as life itself; as an industrial force it was born yesterday. Among the new wave of white-coated scientists, pin-striped businessmen, and the gullible and avid public, biotechnology lacks a sense of context, it lacks roots. This makes it more difficult to plan and shape the future.

We have learned to exploit the gift of nature. Can we surpass what evolution has produced?

Biotechnology in its many forms is likely to impact all sectors of the economy.

In pharmaceuticals new hormones, vaccines, diagnostic tests and drugs will be produced. Old ones will be produced more economically and with a higher level of purity than before. The problems of effective drug delivery to the right target, at the right time, in the right form and at the right dose will see much progress.

In medicine more genetic diseases will be identified and actual correction of diseases will be possible.

In chemicals old reactions will be conducted under gentler conditions leading to lower costs. New compounds, unobserved in nature, will be synthesized.

In electronics, biotechnology will be intimately married to semiconductors through ion selective field effect transistors and chemical field effect transistors. Molecules and whole biological apparatus will be harnessed and used as information storage and processing devices.

In resources recovery, mineral extraction, and beneficiation, an army of bugs will be enrolled for our benefit.

In energy, alcohol, methane and hydrogen will be produced. We will design refineries for biomass and waste and develop a biochemistry paralleling the petrochemistry of today.

In pollution control, molds, yeasts and bacteria will digest our waste and nucleases will attack airborne and waterborne pathogenic viruses.

In cosmetic products, moistening cream, depilating gels, shampooing agents and the like will be based on the new science.

In agriculture and food processing we will see the fixation of nitrogen in organisms not naturally equipped to perform this feat. We expect crispier french fries, jucier tomatoes and timed ripening of fruit. The use of biotechnology in man's foods and drinks will be expanded and diversified. These are not wild predictions. They are only mild projections of current projects and activities. This is not all a dream. A number of products and processes of recombinant DNA technology have been commercially produced: interferon, insulin, human growth hormone, and tissue plasminogen activator.

A recipe for success includes a hope: that government control shall not be burdensome while protecting the interest of the people; that industry will show some social conscience in the selection of commercializable projects and that secrecy shall not starve the burgeoning field; that instruments of destruction by the use of recombinant DNA techniques in chemical and biological warfare shall not be permitted; that the marketplace shall not be manipulated but shall respond to innovations in an orderly fashion; that the investment community shall not be scared by the slow progress; and that the public shall not surrender its right to influence and direct the development of the new technology. That is our dream.

4

Biotechnology and Defense

INTRODUCTION

The possibility of using biotechnology in defense applications has stirred a great deal of interest and controversy. The fundamental research and limited industrial attempts have demonstrated the great potential of the technology. The spector of expanded biological/chemical warfare has filled many with horror.

In this chapter we do not address this controversy with its national security, social, and ethical implications [1,2]. Rather, we present a technological assessment of what has been accomplished and what we can expect in the future [3-6]. The information is organized under broad headings of alarm and detection, chemical/biological warfare, decontamination, medical therapy, energy production, and bioelectronics.

ALARM AND DETECTION

A series of devices has been developed for the detection of cholinesterase inhibitors. Inhibition of the enzyme involved in neuromuscular signal transmission is the primary mode of action of anti-personal agents. The detection principle is as follows: the cholinesterase enzyme is immobilized on some support material, an acetyl choline substrate flows by the membrane and is hydrolyzed to species which are measured electrochemically; introduction of an inhibitor (e.g., CBW agent, organophosphorus pesticides) inhibits the ability of the enzyme to hydrolyze the substrate; the concentration of the inhibitor can be related to the reduced enzyme activity. The detectors used have either been enzyme electrodes, chemical field effect transistors or enzyme thermistors.

Of all the biotechnologies, the production and use of monoclonal antibodies (MAB) is the most rapidly expanding field and is reaching the marketplace faster than any other product. The production of monoclonal (pure clones) antibody is rather simple. An antigen (a foreign substance to an organism) of interest is injected into a mouse. A few days later the mouse's spleen is removed. It contains large amounts of white cells producing antibodies to the antigen injected. These cells are mixed with fast dividing cancer cells—myelomas and a chemical, polyethylene glycol (to effect fusion between the two kinds of cells). The result is an hybridoma. The fusion of the antibody producing cells with the fast dividing cancer cells provides a product retaining both capabilities: virtually dividing forever and producing an endless supply of pure antibodies. The hybridoma is usually kept alive in a mouse which is tapped at regular intervals to retrieve material from which the antibodies are separated. *In vitro* culturing has also been applied to the production of monoclonal antibodies. It is possible to produce MAB against any specific antigen. The specificity, speed, and sensitivity of the antigen antibody reaction make it an ideal detector for complex molecules present in small quantity in a mixture of other chemical species. MAB can be engineered for detecting infectious agents, viruses, cell surface markers, hormones, and chemicals in general. MAB for some 200 antigens are commercially available mostly for research purposes. The detection of the antigen/antibody reaction can be affected with a color reaction (dye), a radioactive marker, an enzyme electrode, or by simply observing agglutination.

The transfer of kits developed for clinical tests to biological/chemical warfare agents detection is a small step. The Chemical Systems Lab of the Army is investigating MAB as a possible alarm and detection system for nerve gas agents; for battlefield applications as well as the protection of workers involved in R&D or production.

It is interesting to postulate other military applications for enzyme based chemical field effect transistors, electrodes and thermistors: the detection of explosives, the identification of chemical leaks, the presence of enemy personnel in a presumed inhabited area, etc. Enzymes in the form of enzyme immunoassays have also been used for drug screenings, an increasing problem in our armed forces. The system, increasingly popular in clinical medicine, is based on an enzyme linked immuno sorbent assay, whereas residual enzyme activity after an immuno reaction is the indicator of drug concentration.

CHEMICAL/BIOLOGICAL WARFARE

The Chemical Systems Laboratory has responsibility for developing chemical warfare agents, incapacitating agents, smoke and obscurants. This array of chemicals is usually classified as nerve agents (GA, GB, VX, VM), incapacitating agents (BZ, EA, EA3839), blister agents (mustard, lewisite), blood agents (cyanide compounds –CK, AC), riot control agents (CN, CS, CR, DM, EA4923), simulants and binary agents. The incapacitating agents of interest are cholinergics, anticholinergics, analgesics, emetics, tranquilizers or anesthetics. The most likely and typical chemical agent to be used under battlefield conditions is an organophosphate agent reacting with the active site of cholinesterase molecules. The biological agents of interest include pathogenic microorganisms (bacteria, viruses, rickettssiae, fungi) and toxins [7,8].

It is difficult to think that man could outwit nature and produce toxins more noxious than what nature had produced by anthrax bacilli. There are obvious ways by recombinant DNA to produce new toxic agents. Their control and their survival outside the laboratory pose such immense problems for limited gain, that it is not believed that the path will be pursued. In this area it is unlikely that biotechnology would produce new ideas and effectively compete against nature with millions of years of practical genetic engineering. On the other hand, biotechnology can do much to improve the characteristics and behavior of organisms and toxins: persistence in the environment, resistance to decontamination agents, timed release, delivery routes, protection of friendly forces, etc.

DECONTAMINATION

In the case of exercise, accident or actual war situation, decontamination must take place prior to personnel reentering the field of action. Most decontaminants under development are water base detergents or surface active agents or reactive neutralizing material (STB, DS2) [7].

Microorganisms and enzymes are diverse. Many specialized cells and catalysts have been isolated that can destroy living organisms and complex chemical entities. Petroleum eating bacteria and microbes which thrive on DDT are already available. Bacteria are used extensively in sewage treatment and in industrial cleanup and decontamination operations. Immobilized ribonuclease can destroy strains of influenza, herpes, and coxsackie viruses. Immobilized peroxidase kills *E. coli* and

Staphylococcus aureus. A packed bed of *Pseudomonas aerucinosa* remove nitrate and dissolved plutonium.

It is easy to extend this work to live organisms and enzyme systems effectively destroying biological and chemical agents at will; providing decontamination of hardware, clothing, water and air.

Fascinating work is being done on developing synthetic or artificial enzymes which perform the enzymatic feats based on a totally or partially engineered catalyst. The hope is to develop cheaper catalysts, less sensitive to the many destructive and inactivating agents (temperature, pH, etc.) or to build catalysts which activate totally new reactions.

As modernization takes place, demilitarization and disposal of toxic material must be built in the cycle. Incineration is the currently favored method. Biological methods would be worth investigating.

MEDICAL THERAPY

The forces of the United States could be called upon at any moment to travel to faraway lands and remain for considerable periods of time. Vaccination has virtually eliminated the threat of epidemics (except maybe for influenza, sexually transmitted diseases and acquired immune deficiency syndrome (AIDS)) in this country. The situation is not comparable in many third world countries. The DOD has interest in developing vaccines (which would be considered orphan drugs by the U.S. pharmaceutical industry) to protect its personnel against little known or rare diseases [3,5].

Conventional virus vaccines are made either from viruses that have been inactivated or from live viruses that have lost their ability to cause the disease. The Salk polio and influenza vaccines are of that inactivated virus type; while the Sabin polio vaccine uses a live organism.

Synthetic vaccines are made of short strings of amino acids that have the shape that a cell surface antibody would recognize. This way they fool the organism to produce antibodies that seek and destroy natural viruses. Recombinant DNA comes into play by identifying the surface antigen gene (say for hepatitis) introducing that gene into another host organism, and inducing it to produce large amounts of the protein of interest.

The industry is at work developing synthetic vaccines against hepatitis, foot and mouth disease, herpes and malaria. The possibility of developing vaccines to fight cancer and a birth control vaccine are real possibilities. The Army is working on vaccines against organisms such as Rickettsia, malaria plasmodium and Rif valley fever agent.

Developments in biotechnology will find many applications in emergency medicine and in the treatment of war wounds: artificial skin, universal donor blood, artificial blood, enzymes for wound debridement, and collagen for aesthetic reconstruction.

ENERGY

The interest of the military on the impact of biotechnology on energy is similar to the nation as a whole with additional constraints such as mobility, reliability and operability under a wide range of conditions, in hostile environments and under special situations such as remote locations, in submarines or aboard ships.

Most of the research has focused on the hydrolysis of starches and cellulosic waste materials to produce alcohol. Interest is growing in bio fuel cell using immobilized enzymes or whole cells (e.g., *Clostridium butyricum*) to produce an electric current upon oxidizing a readily available substrate such as glucose or methanol. Such a device could eventually serve as auxiliary power sources undersea, in outer space, or aboard vessels. Immobilized enzymes have also been used to perform photosynthetic water-splitting, producing hydrogen [6].

BIOELECTRONICS

It is the concensus of most experts that current methods of fabricating semiconductors will reach fundamental limits, in terms of packing density, after only a few more doublings. Also, high density increases the proportion of defective chips and packaging and inspection cost increase dramatically with density. The current status is about 2^{16} transistors per chip, a line width of 2.5 μm, a power dissipation in the range of 0.1–0.2 mW and a cost of 0.002 cent per bit for memory units. Improvements are likely to occur with focused electron beams replacing ultraviolet and x-ray in lithography, and progress in three dimensional microelectronic devices.

Recently, the new field of molecular electronics was born. Its aim is to replace the transistor with organic or inorganic molecular functional groups exhibiting similar behavior.

Several research groups are hard at work on anisotropic materials: organo-metallic charge-transfer complexes, conductive organic polymers, and biological polymers as electronic switching devices. These complexes display unusual, potentially important and useful behavior when exposed to electric currents or high intensity light. They are capable of storing information in erasable form and to act as semi-conductors. The name biotic has been proposed, by analogy with robotic, for the new technology attempting to marry biology and information science.

Two promising avenues are being pursued. One is based on harnessing biological micro-apparatus behaving like diodes. The other building upon soliton (a mathematical concept akin to a wave) behavior in conductive polymers.

The material of most interest is trans-polyactylene, a polymer consisting of a zig-zagging carbon chain with alternating single and double bonds. When two such chains, organized in opposite direction of zig-zagging, meet; the boundary between the chains can move along the chain, that is the soliton can propagate along the chain. When three such chains meet at a point, we have a switch, the soliton moving down one or the other chain depending on the pattern of double bonds. Moreover, when the soliton has passed, it changes the patterns of bonds.

Another chemical diode recently reported is made of an electron donor (tetrathiosulfalene (TTF)), in insulating bridge (urethane) and an electron acceptor (tetracyanoquinodimethane (TCNQ)). This switch can be driven by electric current or by laser light in less than 5 nanoseconds.

A number of small biological structures can be harnessed as switches or memory elements. The cytochrome electron transport system is one such system. Other examples include the photosynthetic apparatus and microtobules in nervous system cells with a density of 10^{15} elements/mm^2.

Ultimately, and this is where biotechnology really comes into play, it should be possible to use the capacity for auto assembly present in biological macromolecules. Great strides have been made by designing machines that can use this self-assembly processing in synthesizing a gene based on a man-made program. A similar process might be employed in fabricating a molecular logic device composed of self-assembling protein components. Ironically, a combination of computer aided design and recombinant DNA technology will be required to specify and then synthesize (by programmed microorganisms) the protein subunits.

Most of the work is theoretical, but the possibility exists to build, over the next 20 to 50 years a biochemical computer. Such an eventual computer will pack tremendous storage capacity and computing power in the tiniest volume. Achieving this goal will require not only advances in the development of biomolecular components, but radical departures from conventional computer architecture (a sixth or seventh generation computer, perhaps).

A formidable "silicon wall" exists today in terms of the gap between conventional microelectronics and unconventional bioelectronics. But an information revolution is taking place—sometimes closer to science fiction than reality, sometimes based on sound theories and practices.

ESOTERICA

Secret Codes

DNA (deoxyribonucleic acid) is a long twisted double helix of alternating bases on a backbone of sugar with phosphate binding groups. The sequence of the four bases: adenine (A), guanine (G), thymine (T) and cytosine (C) is the essential message directing the cell machinery to produce specific proteins which are the basis for all the biochemistry. A four letter sequence—this is a code. It is possible to use such a linear sequence as a coding scheme for transmitting secret information.

The neat idea would be to create such a code and to insert it in a living cell, lost in the long DNA sequence of the cell; it would remain undetected except to the intended recipient knowing where to look.

- We understand the structure of the DNA and its four bases organized in a sequence.
- We appreciate the fundamental dogma of biology: the DNA in the nucleus is transcribed into a messenger RNA which migrate to the cytoplasm and is read by ribosomes which manufacture proteins with the help of the transfer RNA's.
- We visualize the protein as a sequence made up of 20 different amino acids sequence. Beyond that, folding and shape give the protein its binding capacity, selectivity and activity.

This is a simple process with great possibilities. For example, how many different sequences of 100 amino acids can be built out of 20 different amino acids: 20^{100}. The possibilities are mind-boggling.

Genetic engineering is not that complex (Figure 4-1). Three basic steps are involved: 1) the isolation of the desired DNA region; 2) the insertion of the isolated donor DNA fragment into a vector genome; 3) the growth and multiplication of the vector in a host organism.

The process of creating a DNA message involves starting with a well defined messenger RNA (the message), then to reverse the normal process and create a complementary double stranded DNA. Next, it is

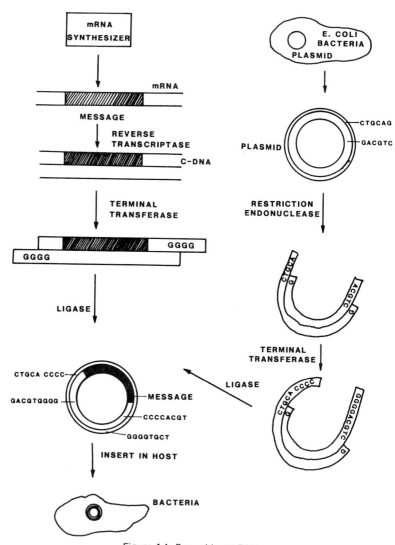

Figure 4-1. Recombinant DNA.

necessary to give it sticky ends. And lastly, to merge the strands in the awaiting hole in a suitably prepared plasmid. The insertion of the plasmid in the host bacteria completes the trick.

The system would have to have two keys: 1) the specific set of restriction enzymes, the endonucleases, used for cutting the right piece of DNA containing the message, and, 2) a code or a dictionary based on a four-letter alphabet.

Four letters is a rather poor alphabet. Why not copy nature and use a linear, comma free, non-overlapping triplet code. Four bases, taken three at a time equals 64 words. A very decent dictionary allowing for the 26 letters of the alphabet, the ten digits and special symbols.

System complexity can be enhanced almost at will by learning from nature. Reading could be done in the three possible frames with overlapping messages. The message could be made of exons separated by introns in the DNA and would require transcription to mRNA prior to decoding. Garbage DNA could be introduced at will throughout the sequence. All information required for decoding could be inserted in the form of sequences (inverted, inverted repeats, palindromes, etc.) in the header.

For sure, the coding density of such a system is not attractive. Its advantage is more associated with the fact that the code can be lost in an ocean to DNA, it is much smaller than a microdot and the host organism can be easily carried in the intestine of a human.

Enzymatic Screening

We, today, know of thousands of "genetic diseases" and we increasingly are realizing that psychological diseases such as drug addiction, schizophrenia, etc., are chemically (hence enzymatically) mediated. The concept of screening U.S. workers to detect propensity or sensitivity to adverse environments has raised important ethical and legal issues. Essentially a worker might be denied the possibility of earning higher wages because of an enzymatic quirk.

The effectiveness of our Armed Forces depends on no other factor more than the quality of the personnel. It is possible to forecast the day when enzymatic screening will rival with medical and psychological tests in defining the health of people as well as predicting their behavior under stress or hostile environmental conditions.

CONCLUSION

Over the next 20 years biotechnology is likely to impact on war doctrine, personnel selection and training and actual combat operations. The key developments are not likely to be in the development of new biological agents or toxins, but in better methods of detection, protection and decontamination. Peripheral functions (of the infrastructure type), in the conduct of war, such as energy and medicine are the major targets for important biotechnology breakthroughs. The Department of

Defense (DOD) is very much like a country. It is a state in itself. It has a large work force. Its budget is larger than the gross national product of many countries. It has extensive contract and specification authority. In many parts of the country it drives the local economy. To satisfy its mission, DOD maintains a sophisticated fabrication and manufacturing capability. It consumes vast amounts of energy and has a sophisticated medical establishment. In other words, it is a microcosm of the U.S. and most modern countries. This has led the DOD to erect a substantial infrastructure. Many of the biotechnology interests of DOD will be in support of this infrastructure: energy production, environmental protection, medical assurance and health maintenance.

REFERENCES

1. Wagner, R. L. and T. S. Gould, "Why We Can't Avoid Developing Chemical Weapons," *Defense, 82,* 3–11 (July 1982).
2. Zamparutti, T., "Baltimore on Genetic Research: Future Possibilities and Ethical Questions Remain," *MIT Report,* 6-1-83 (1983).
3. Hiam, A., "Military Genetic Engineering Reconsidered," *Genetic Engineering News,* 4 (Jan/Feb 1983).
4. Zochlinski, "Army DNA Researchers Try to Shed Bio-Warrior Image," *Genetic Engineering News,* 31 (Sept/Oct 1982).
5. Zochlinski, "Biotechnology in Military R&D: Two Firms Look for Future Profits in Joint Projects," *Genetic Engineering News,* 4 (Jan/Feb 1983).
6. Findl, E., H. Gutherman, and J. Johnsen, "Immobilized Enzymes/Bacteria for Naval Applications," Initial Data Base, Office of Naval Research AD-AC 98801 (1981).
7. Harris, B. L., "Chemical Warfare—A Primer," *ChemTech,* 2–35 (January 1982).
8. Lovelace, G. M., "Chemical Warfare," *Nato's Fifteen Nations,* 54–56 (Dec. 1981–Jan. 1982).

5

Biotechnology and the Food and Agricultural Sector

INTRODUCTION

B *iotechnology has been* heralded as the key to a new age. It promises crops resistant to drought, and insect and disease free; a less energy intensive agriculture and a lessened dependence on synthetic fertilizer; the management of problem weeds and pests without dangerous chemicals; increased yield in traditional crops and the introduction of new food crops. How many of these promises can be realized is the subject of this review.

A variety of techniques are simultaneously attacking secular problems in the agricultural sector with a new vigor: in-vitro fertilization, cell culture, regeneration of transformed plants, induced mutations, plant tissue and embryo culture, genetic hybridization, sex control, protoplast cell fusion, and the build-up of germ plasm stocks.

Biotechnology is the newest technique to be applied to solving the basic agricultural challenges:

- increase crops yield by incorporating resistance to drought, pests, etc. These factors claim up to 20% of the annual crop yield.
- improve the nutritional value of crops, especially missing amino acids;
- lower the production cost by eliminating the need for chemical fertilization and the use of chemical pesticides.

The plant kingdom is vast. A number of actions, based on biotechnologies, could be taken to improve the way we grow and use plants for food. A limited set will be reviewed either because solving the problem would have dramatic social and economic impact, or because near term solutions are in the offerings.

55

Action potential	Time frame
Photosynthesis improvement	15-20 yrs
Resistance to disease, pests, etc.	1-4 yrs
Nitrogen fixation	15 yrs
Plant improvement	
Hybridization	now
Gene transfer	1-4 yrs
Cloroplast fusion	1-4 yrs

THE LIMIT TO PHOTOSYNTHESIS

The efficiency of the photosynthetic process is around 1%. Can biotechnology improve on nature's low efficiency? The basic climatic limitation to crop photosynthesis is the seasonal input of light energy as modified by local climatic factors such as temperature, water, etc. The length of the growing season is therefore a limitation on crop yield [1].

Many have lamented on the photorespiratory loss and have postulated possible mechanisms for limiting such losses. The pineapple plant, for instance, can produce a given amount of dry weight with 7-10 times less waste loss than corn or rice [2]. Is it possible to transfer this metabolic characteristic to c_3 plants?

At a more fundamental level, the ribulose biphosphate carboxylase/oxygenase enzyme system is the point of entry of carbon into the Benson-Calvin cycle, and of oxygen in the photorespiratory pathway. It is a pivotal point in the overall efficiency of the photosynthetic system. The possibility of acting on the genetic system is made very difficult by the existence of two interacting genetic control systems; one found in the choloplast, the other in the cytoplasm.

It has been estimated that photosynthetic efficiency could be improved from 1 to 3 to 5 percent by [3]:

• improving the efficiency of the photosynthetic collector system;
• increasing the efficiency of the energy use, once absorbed by the photosynthetic pigment;
• partitioning the product of the dark reactions of photosynthesis.

About 90 percent of the dry weight of plants is derived from photosynthesis. The genes involved in carbon fixation are only now being elucidated. Eventually it should be possible to act directly on genes involved in photorespiration, carboxylation, electron transport, and translocation of photosynthetic products.

Plant life is a rather inefficient chemical system. It is theoretically possible to redesign such a system to improve its efficiency and productivity [4]:

- *Reduction in the amount of DNA*—The chloroplast and mitochondria genome contains many multiple copies. No role has been found for this "junk" DNA. An energy cost is associated with its duplication. If this DNA is truly non-functional, its elimination would improve plant productivity by saving the energy involved.
- *Minimization of respiratory losses*—A very large amount of fixed CO_2 is lost in photorespiration. The ability to minimize photorespiration (achieved in certain plants, especially C_4) represents an enormous potential for productivity enhancement.
- *Conservation of seed germination energy*—Much energy is involved in the synthesis of enzymes involved in mobilizing seed reserves. Minimizing this process to the essential level only, would make more energy available for growth.
- *Reduction in foliage*—Considerable energy is expanded in the production and maintenance of surplus foliage. The reduction of such foliage by altering the leaf morphology and limiting their area would enhance productivity.

A FIXATION FOR NITROGEN

Plants need nitrogen to make amino acids, the building blocks of all proteins. Cereals such as corn and rice cannot use nitrogen from the air. Costly chemically fixed nitrogen must be used. U.S. farmers apply about 19 kg of nitrogen per hectare. 40 million BTUs are required to produce one ton of ammonia. 5.9×10^{14} BTUs or the energy equivalent of 100 million barrels of crude oil are invested in making ammonia for nitrogen fertilizer [5-11].

Legumes, on the other hand, are infected by symbiotic bacteria from the genus *Rhizobium*, capable of using energy supplied by the plants to convert nitrogen to ammonia. A number of free living nitrogen fixing bacteria (*Klebsiella, Azotobacter, Clostridium, Rhodospirillum, Asperillum*), and cyanobacteria reduce nitrogen for their own use [12].

A number of strategies are possible:

- adapt naturally occurring associations between nitrogen fixing soil bacteria and the roots of cereal plants;
- genetically modify both rhizobial species and cereals so that a true symbiotic relationship can be established;

- improve the efficiency of the nitrogen fixing system;
- transfer bacterial nitrogen fixing genes to plants.

NIF

The nif gene complex contains 17 different genes. Three of these genes make the proteins that combine to make up the nitrogenase enzyme. The location of the nif operon including structural, regulatory and cofactors genes has been determined for *Klebsiella pneunomiae*. The nif gene has been transferred by recombinant DNA techniques among microbes [12]. The challenge is to transfer such a system to higher plants.

The possibility exists to construct, in vitro, a genetic vehicle carrying nitrogen fixation genes capable of crossing the prokaryotic-eukaryotic barriers of DNA uptake.

Many laboratories are at work in [13]:

- developing a package of engineered nitrogen fixation genes;
- defining a vector for carrying the package into plants; and
- developing a suitable biochemical environment within plant cells where nitrogen fixation can occur.

HUP

One factor limiting the efficiency of symbiotic nitrogen fixation is the release of hydrogen during the nitrogenase reaction. About 25 to 30% of the energy in the nitrogen fixing system is lost as hydrogen gas. The most efficient strains have an hup (hydrogen uptake) system capable of oxidizing the hydrogen, and thus preventing the energy loss. The hup system (since it uses oxygen to oxidize the hydrogen) also protects the oxygen-sensitive nitrogenase enzyme from inactivation. *Rhizobium* that have a hup system have a higher nitrogenase activity. Soybeans innoculated with hup-containing strains produce 16 percent higher yield than soybeans innoculated with organisms without the hydrogen uptake system [14].

SYM

The sym (for symbiosis) plasmid identified in *Rhizobium trifolii* seems to recognize and infect the appropriate host. The possibility exists to transfer this gene to other organisms.

The Market

In 1980, over $10 billion was spent on fertilizers and soil conditioners, or about $4200 per farm [14]. It is estimated that the worldwide demand for fertilizer nitrogen will grow to 200 million tons annually by the year 2000, based on current usage [13]. These numbers provide an economic incentive for the experimental work underway.

PLANT IMPROVEMENT

Over the last 10,000 years, man has used some 3,000 species of plants. About 150 species have entered into commerce. The world population is today fed by about 15 species of plants (rice, wheat, corn, sorghum, barley, common bean, soybean, peanut, potato, sweet potato, cassava, sugar cane, sugar beet, coconut, banana) [15].

For sure, great improvements have been achieved by traditional techniques: hybridization (the green revolution is a good example if you can wait for a 12-year program of breeding and selection) [16], fertilizers (vegetables may out yield wild relatives by 100 times) [17], pesticides, etc. Many unexploited species remain and the possibility of finding new crops adapted for production on marginal land is a real option [18].

The importance of protein quality, digestibility and utilization in food is rapidly being recognized. Legumes are especially nutritionally deficient in sulpho amino acids. This is important since in certain parts of the world, they are the main source of proteins. Several attempts have been made to incorporate high lyzine in maize, barley and sorghum. Success has been forthcoming with some reduction in yield [19].

Gene Transfer

Hybridization has improved by a factor of four the per acre yield of corn in the last 50 years. Similar claims can be made for other crops. Breeding is a costly, time-consuming trial and error method dealing only with qualities already in the seed. Genetic engineering is, in principle, permitting to tap an almost unlimited gene pool from animals and plants. This promising technique is the transferring of genes. The progress has been slow because of the lack of a good vector. This was the situation until the idea of introducing the desired genetic material by linking it to a highly invasive vector came to the surface. The TI (Tumor-inducing) plasmid of the bacteria *Agrobacterium tumefaciens* is a good candidate [20,21]. Scientists at Monsanto and at the University of Ghent have been successful in inserting a bacterial gene into plants [22,23].

Although geneticists have transferred many genes via TI plasmids in higher plants, in most cases the trait is not expressed in the mature plant. A very nice exception is a factor moved into tobacco cells by Cetus scientists and grown for three generations. The basic problem here is the need to carry with the gene of interest its proper genetic control signals.

Other vector or delivery systems being tested include the cauliflower mosaic virus (CMV) and the root-inducing (RI) plasmid from *A. Rhizogenes* [24–28].

Eventually many new traits will be incorporated into and expressed in higher plants. The real possibility exists to engineer totally new plants.

Cell Fusion

Protoplasts can easily be isolated from leaf tissues, cultured cells, and other sources. The first step in cell fusion is the digestion of the cell wall by enzymes. The fusion process is mediated through the use of polyethylene glycol. A number of hybrid cell combinations have been reported covering many plant species and families [29–31].

soybean + barley
carrot + barley
tobacco + soybean
potato + tomatoe
carrot + parsley
sorghum + corn
clover + soybean
corn + soybean
alfalfa + soybean
rapeseed + soybean

Mutants

Cell cultures can be a source of spontaneous or induced mutants with interesting traits [32]. One basic difficulty with spontaneous mutations is its low rate, about 1×10^{-5} per gene copy per year. Unfortunately few spontaneous mutants of potential agriculture use have been isolated this way. New methods for selecting cellular mutants are needed. The most important problem is probably associated with the mutant phenotype retention in regenerated plants. A number of well established techniques are available for inducing mutation. These methods increase the mutation rate and hence the chance of detecting a useful mutant.

RESISTANCE

Intensive programs of genetic engineering are under way to improve resistance to cold, blight, insects; speed maturation, improve solid content (tomatoes); and insure resistance to drought, salt and flooding [33].

Water Resistance

Increased salinity in soil is causing farmers $32 million/year in reduced crop yield in the San Joaquin valley alone. Some nations, such as India and Australia, are largely arid or semi-arid zones demanding plants capable of living under salt and low moisture conditions.

Efficient use of water is the clear goal of all dry land agriculture systems [34]. Breeders have occasionally selected extensive rooting plants to achieve higher yields under moisture stress [35]. The traditional approach to insuring resistance to drought is the development of cultivars with greater water use efficiency. The probability of selecting such a system by present breeding methods is infinitesimally small [36]. More promising would be to identify the gene associated with water use efficiency [37].

OSM is the osmoregulatory gene. High salt content in soil creates high osmotic pressure, hence reducing the availability of soil water to plants. A set of genes exists in many plants and bacteria cells to prevent water loss. In principle it should be possible to isolate and transfer this gene to give salt tolerance capability to higher plants [12].

Frosty the Bacterium

Frost injury causes millions of dollars in crop damage every year in the United States to corn, soybeans, wheat, and citrus fruits, as well as potatoes. It is well known that certain bacteria produce nuclei for ice crystal formation and help produce frost damage when the temperature drops below the freezing point of water. A scientist at the University of California after identifying the DNA fragment responsible, snipped it out with endonuclease enzymes. The bacteria can now be released without fear of frost damage. Field tests are underway to document the effectiveness of the technique.

Pesticide Resistance

Pesticides are poisons designed to kill pests and problem weeds. Two problems arise with extensive use of pesticides: they more often than not affect unintended species, and the targets develop resistance or tolerance over time. A new problem recently observed is the accelerated degradation of certain pesticides by soil organisms. This degradation is sometimes so rapid that the product loses its efficacy. The pesticides affected by accelerated breakdown by microbes are the carbofuran insecticides and the thiocarbamate herbicides. While biodegradation is a desirable property; a fine balance must be maintained between efficacy and accumulation in the food chain [38].

A total of over 200 examples of resistance are known and some pests are escaping our ability to control them with chemicals [39]. For instance, resistance to triazine has been documented in at least 17 genera and 26 species of weeds [40].

A number of new lines of crops tolerant to herbicides have been developed. Notable is a new line of corn developed by Molecular Genetics and Cyanamid. The major impact of such new lines is to increase the market for broad-spectrum herbicides which otherwise would have limited potential with current hybrids of corn [41].

A mutant-bacteria gene that confers resistance to the broad spectrum glycosate has been discovered at Calgene. If inserted in crops, the gene would enable farmers to use more phosphone methylglycine for problem weeds control [42].

In a similar effort, scientists at Michigan State University found that a single change in a choloplast gene can account for the development of resistance to the herbicide atrazine in certain weeds. The incorporation of such a gene in soybeans is the next likely target [43].

Biopesticides

Biopesticides are natural pathogens, and pests cannot develop resistance to them. Bacterial, viral, and fungal agents are applicable to above ground pests. Nematodes and protozoa products should be possible for controlling soil inhabiting organisms [44].

Bacteria

Bacteria as pesticides have received the most attention, especially *Bacillus thurengiensis* which is effective against more than 100 species of lepidoptera. Manufacturers are developing new formulations to protect bacterial insecticides against environmental deactivating forces. While the bacillus has been used in the agricultural arena; nothing prevents from using it against carriers of diseases such as mosquitoes and flies.

The bacillus kill pests by releasing toxic crystals in the gut of the larvae having ingested it. The genes encoding the cyrstal producing system are carried on plasmids. *Bacillus subtilis* might be an appropriate host for cloning the gene.

Viruses

Baculoviruses can cause diseases in insects. Viral bioinsecticides can be produced by growing them in host insects or in tissue culture. A number of industrial products (e.g., Elcar, Gypcheck) are on the market; more are being developed and tested.

Fungi

Fungi as bioinsecticides can be readily mass produced by fermentation. Their tendency to produce air-borne spores that cause allergy is a limiting factor. *Bovaria abacerna* has been used for aphid control. More candidates are being worked on.

Nematodes and Protozoas

Nematodes and protozoas are interesting candidates for in-ground pests. These specialized pesticides will fill a vacuum in the pesticide arsenal.

Plant Vaccines

The possibility to induce resistance by increasing defenses against virus and bacteria is not limited to human and animals. Induced resistance is taking place in natural population every day. Interest is growing in plant vaccines, in the form of spray or as part of fertilizer, containing enough pathogen to induce resistance in future generation.

Allelopathic Chemicals

A war is going on between plants and between plants and insects. So far the plants are winning. These plants involved in a merciless chemical warfare use a wide range of toxic chemicals called allelopathic. These chemicals are volatilized from leaves, leaches from leaves or litter, and exuded from roots. These chemicals include amino acids and their alcohols, simple lactones, quinones, flavonoids, tannins, alkaloids, terpenes, and steroids. Their modes of action are equally varied: stimulation or inhibition of respiration, photosynthesis inhibition, effect on protein synthesis, alteration of the permeability of membranes, inhibition of germination, the degradation of cell walls in plants, and inhibition of plant enzymes [45,46]. Some of these chemical defense systems are very ingenious. For instance, some chemicals such as furano coumarins are toxic only when the insects (having ingested the chemicals) are exposed to light [46,47].

The Market

The pesticide market in the U.S. is of the order of $3.25 billion. The market for chemicals used to formulate agricultural pesticides will grow 16 percent by 1987 to $245 million. The breakdown is as follows [48]:

Surfactants, adjuvants	$110	45%
Solvents	54	22
Diluents, carriers	47	19
Others (deactivators, thickeners, antifoams, etc.)	34	14

FOOD PROCESSING

Our review so far has concentrated on producing food. Food processing, in a health and nutrition conscious society demanding services of every kind, is a critical step in the food chain.

Enzymes

Enzymes are used in food processing mainly for economic reasons. Where they are used (and the market is relatively small) they perform functions difficult or more expensive to accomplish by other means. Rennin, essential to the cheese making process represents half of this market [49]. A rapidly-growing market are the enzymes involved in the production of high fructose corn syrup.

Most enzymes used in food processing are crude extracts. Important efforts are underway to clone such enzyme systems in bacteria and to improve the required purification process. For example, the gene for pre-pro-rennin has been cloned in *E. coli* by Collaborative Research, Inc.

Important progresses will be made in the near future in using a wider range of specialized enzymes in food processing; and in improving the performance of existing enzymes through immobilization and structural modifications.

Single Cell Proteins

If plants and animals are not enough or too expensive, how shall we feed the growing world? One possibility is the production of single cell proteins from inexpensive raw material.

Diverse strains of organism (*Pseudomonads, Aspergillus niger, Methylopholus methylotropus, Candida utilis, Chaetomium cellulolyticum*), metabolic substrates (molasses, methane, methanol, n-paraffins, biological wastes), and fermentation equipment have been tested in the laboratory, pilot plant, and in commercial operations around the world [50–53].

Single cell proteins have now been produced for some 20 years on a relatively small scale. The better known processes are:

ICI	"Pruteen"
Phillips Petroleum	"Provesteen"
Waterloo/Enviricon	

In this field the British are the leaders. Plants have also been built in the U.S., Italy, Canada, Spain, France, Rumania, Germany, and Venezuela to mention a few cases. In Russia, an aggressive single cell protein program is pursued by the State to help alleviate chronic food shortages [54].

Some of the impediments associated with an expanded SCP market are its energy requirements [55], its contents in nucleic acids, its texture, and its behavior during cooking.

Genetic engineering has been used to improve the efficiency of the basic *Methylophilus methylotropus* organism in the ICI process. Basically the glutamate synthetase producing gene has been mutated inactivating it (improving nitrogen assimilation) and an hydrogenase gene extracted from *E. coli* was inserted in the organism [56].

Protein additives are close to a $700 million market. Soybean derived proteins, whey derived proteins, and yeast proteins are the major sources [57].

CONCLUSIONS

Plant cells contain as many as 100,000 genes, few of which have been identified as to their function, location and sequence [58]. Our knowledge of plants biochemicals pathways and molecular biology is limited making the application of techniques successful in microbiology more problematic [59].

First successes of biotechnology in the agricultural sector will be associated with manipulating monogenic traits associated with resistance. Agricultural losses due to insects, pests, diseases, and weeds prior to harvesting total about $10 billion (the actual U.S. harvest annual value is estimated at $25 billion). This represents a technical and economic challenge to biotechnology.

The problems of nitrogen fixation and photosynthetic improvement will be longer to solve but the payback will be phenomenal.

Agriculture exports amount to some $45 billion, helping our balance of payment situation. It is expected that the systematic and intelligent application of biotechnology will contribute substantially to maintaining our leadership.

REFERENCES

1. Foyer, C., R. Leegoud, and D. Walker, "What Limits Photosynthesis?" *Nature, 298,* 326 (1982).

2. Bonner, J., "The Application of Genetic Engineering to Agriculture, The World's Largest and Oldest Industry," in *Genetic Engineering, International Conference,* April 6–10, 1981, Reston, Va., Batelle Memorial Institute (1981).

3. Miles, C. D., "Genetic of Photosynthesis," in *Genetic Engineering, Intl. Conf.,* April 6–10, Reston, Va., Battelle Memorial Institute (1981).

4. Rao, A. S. and R. Singh, "Theoretical Approaches for Reducing Bioenergetic Costs and Enhancing Plant Productivity," *J. Theor. Biol., 104,* 113–120 (1983).

5. Brill, W. J., "Nitrogen Fixation: Basic to Applied," *Amer. Scientist, 676* (4), 458–466 (1979).

6. "Nitrogen Fixation Research Advances," *C&EN,* 29–30 (Dec. 8, 1980).

7. Marx, J. L., "Nitrogen Fixation: Prospects for Genetic Manipulation," *Science, 196,* 638–641 (1977).

8. Evans, H. J. and A. L. E. Barber, "Bilogical Nitrogen Fixation for Food and Fiber Production," *Science, 197,* 332–339 (1977).

9. Shanmugam, K. T. and R. C. Valentine, "Molecular Biology of Nitrogen Fixation," *Science, 187,* 919–924 (1975).

10. Safrany, D. R., "Nitrogen Fixation," *Sci. Amer.,* 64–80.

11. Skinner, K. J., "Nitrogen Fixation," *C&EN, 4,* 27–35 (1976).

12. Kidd, G. H., M. E. Davis, and P. Esmailzadeh, "Assessment of Future Environmental Trends and Problems: Agricultural Use of Applied Genetics and Biotechnologies," EPA 600/8-81-019 (1981).

13. Ausubel, F. M., "Nitrogen Fixation," in *Genetic Engineering, International Conference,* April 6–10, 1981, Reston, Va., Battelle Memorial Institute (1981).

14. Marx, J., "Can Crops Grow Without Added Fertilizer?" *High Technology,* 67–69 (March/April 1983).

15. Hall, T. C. and J. D. Kemp, "Enhancing Protein Quality and Quantity," in *Genetic Engineering, International Conf.*, April 6–10, 1981, Reston, Va., Battelle Memorial Institute (1981).

16. Swaminathan, M. S., "Biotechnology Research and Third World Agriculture," *Science, 218,* 967–972 (1982).

17. Tudge, C., "The Future of Crops," *New Scientist,* 547–553 (May 26, 1983).

18. Boyer, J. S., "Plant Productivity and Environment," *Science, 218,* 443–447 (1982).

19. Boulter, D., "Breeding for Protein Yield and Quality," *Nature, 256,* 168–169 (1975).

20. Expert, D., A. Goldman, and J. Tournevr, "Le Crown-Gall: Une Manipulation Genetique Naturelle," *La Recherche, 108,* 212–214 (1980).

21. Marx, J. L., "Crown Gall Disease: Nature as Genetic Engineer," *Science, 203,* 254–255 (1979).

22. De Young, G., "Crop Energetics: The Seeds of Revolution," *High Technology,* 53–59 (June 1983).

23. "Bacterial Gene is Expressed in Cultured Tobacco Cells," *Genetic Engineering News, 3,* 1 (1983).

24. Chilton, M.-D., "A Vector for Introducing New Genes into Plants," *Sci. Amer., 248* (6), 51–59 (1983).

25. Estrella, L.-H., A. Depkker, M. Van Montago, and J. Schell, "Expression of Chimeric Genes Transformed into Plant Cells Using a TI-Plasmid Derived Vector," *Nature, 303,* 209–213 (1983).

26. Bevan, M., "*Agrobacterium tumefaciens* Tumor-Inducing Plasmids as Genetic Engineering Vectors in Plants," in *Genetic Engineering, Int. Conf.,* April 6–10, 1981, Reston, Va., Battelle Memorial Institute (1981).

27. Davies, R., "Gene Transfer in Plants," *Nature, 291,* 531–532 (1981).

28. Drummond, M., "Launching Genes Across Phylogenetic Barriers," *Nature, 303,* 198–199 (1983).

29. Gamborg, O., "New Hybrid Plants," in *Genetic Engineering, Intl. Conf.,* April 6–10, 1981, Reston, Va., Battelle Memorial Institute (1981).

30. Sheppard, J. F., "The Regeneration of Potatoe Plants from Leaf-cell Protoplasts," *Sci. Amer., 246* (5), 154–166 (1982).

31. Cocking, E. C., M. R. Davey, D. Pental, and J. B. Power, "Aspects of Plant Genetic Manipulation," *Nature, 293,* 265–270 (1981).

32. Nabors, M. W., "Using Spontaneously Occurring and Induced Mutations to Obtain Agriculturally Useful Plants," *Bioscience, 26* (12), 761–767 (1976).

33. Williams, P. Y., "Genetic Resistance in Plants," *Genetics, 79,* 409–419 (1975).

34. Reitz, L. P., "Breeding for Efficient Water Use—Is It Real or a Mirage?" *Agri. Meteor., 14,* 3–11 (1974).

35. Hurd, E. A., "Phenotype and Drought Tolerance in Wheat," *Agri. Meteor, 14,* 39–55 (1974).

36. Eslick, R. F. and E. A. Hockett, "Genetic Engineering as a Key to Water-Use Efficiency," *Agri. Meteor., 14,* 13–23 (1974).

37. Moss, D. N., J. T. Woolley, and J. F. Stone, "Plant Modification for More Efficient Water Use: The Challenge," *Agri. Meteor., 14,* 311–320 (1974).

38. Fox, J. L., "Soil Microbes Pose Problems for Pesticides," *Science, 221,* 1029–1031 (1983).

39. Murphy, S. R., "Bioengineering in Agriculture Pesticides," in *Potential Application of Recombinant DNA and Genetics on Agricultural Science,* Hearing before the Subcommittee on Investigation and Oversight, 97th Congress, June 9, 1982, NO. 134 (1982).

40. LeBaron, H. M., "Applications of Herbicide Resistance," in *Genetic Engineering, International Conference,* April 6–10, 1981, Reston, Va., Battelle Memorial Institute (1981).

41. "Agrichemicals," *Chemical Week,* 17 (Oct. 5, 1983).

42. "A Herbicide-Resistant Gene is Developed," *Chemical Week,* 28 (July 27, 1983).

43. Marx, J. L., "Plant's Resistance to Herbicide Pinpointed," *Science, 220,* 41–42 (1983).

44. Lawless, E. W., et al., "A Technology Assessment of Biological Substitutes for Chemical Pesticides," NSF/RA-770508 (1977).

45. Putman, A. R., "Allelopathic Chemicals," *C&EN,* 34–45 (April 4, 1983).

46. Maugh, T. H., II, "Explaining Plant Resistance to Insects," *Science, 216,* 722–723 (1982).

47. *Inside R&D,* 2 (April 14, 1982).

48. "The Coming Revolution in Agricultural Chemicals," *Chemical Week,* 722–723 (June 15, 1983).

49. Whitaker, J. R., "Some Present and Future Uses of Enzymes in the Food Industry," in *Enzymes—The Interface Between Technology and Economics,* J. P. Danehy and B. Wolnak, eds., Marcel Dekker, Inc., New York (1980).

50. Joglekar, R., R. Clerman, R. P. Ouellette, and P. N. Cheremisinoff. *Biotechnology in Industry.* Ann Arbor Science, Ann Arbor, MI (1983).

51. "The New Technology of Single Cell Proteins," *Chemical Week* (1983).

52. Chowdhury, J., "Nonpolluting Process Turn Methanol into Pure Protein," *Chemical Engineering,* 56–57 (Sept. 5, 1983).

53. "Petroproteins: Commercial Answer to Malthus," *Chem. Mark. Rept.,* 16–20 (Feb. 11, 1980).

54. "Russians Catch the Nu-Food Bug," *New Scientist* (May 26, 1983).

55. Lewis, C. W., "Energy Requirements for Single Cell Protein Production," *J. Appl. Chem. Biotech., 26,* 568–575 (1975).

56. "Genetic Engineering Improves SCP Bacteria," *C&EN,* 30 (May 5, 1980).

57. "Food Markets Pick Up for Protein Additives," *Chemical Week,* 36 (Aug. 1, 1979).

58. Solomon, S., "Plants that Break the Gene Barriers," *Science Digest,* 16–30 (April 1983).

59. Cheremisinoff, P. N. and R. P. Ouellette, eds. *Biotechnology: Applications and Research.* Technomic Publishing Co., Inc., Lancaster, PA; Basel, Switz. (1985).

6

Biotechnology and Chemicals

INTRODUCTION

There are an estimated 63,000 chemicals in common use in the United States. On February 24, 1983, *Chemical Abstract* listed its six-millionth chemical. Chemicals are essential to our industrial society. The desire to produce an increasing variety of chemicals by the least expensive and least energy intensive route is stimulating a renewed interest in the use of enzymes, cells, and organisms to achieve these goals.

Microorganisms are known to produce, in small quantities, some 200 chemical substances of commercial value. By 1977, more than 145 companies were using fermentation for the production of fine chemicals, fermentation products as starting materials for chemical synthesis, and therapeutics [1].

At one time or another, the following chemicals have been produced by fermentation [1].

Comenic acid	Butanol
Erythorbic Acid	Glycerol
Gluconic acid	Acetone
Itaconic acid	2,3 butanediol
2-keto-D-gluconic	Vitamins with growth factors
lactic acid	nucleosides and nucleotides
malic acid	amino acids
urocanic acid	polysaccharides
acetic acid	pharmaceuticals (e.g., antibiotics, steroids)
citric acid	enzymes
Ethanol	fragrances and flavors

The list of fermentation processes that have been reviewed is growing; the list of fermentation processes that never made it to commercial scale is much larger. It is important to get at the root of such successes and failures.

The humble bacteria, *E. coli*, is the best known microorganism. Some 3,000 to 6,000 different types of molecules are present in this organism. We have probably unraveled the metabolic pathway for about a third of these reactions. The metabolic pattern of this organism is not substantially different than that found in other organisms and thus can serve as a model. In spite of a diversity of chemicals in living organisms, the basic pathway is surprisingly similar for all living systems (Figure 6-1).

A number of claims have been made about the possibility of producing a number of chemicals by biological routes from a variety of biological raw materials and wastes [2-7].

On the surface, biotechnology for chemicals production appears attractive. Promise of:

• the use of renewable resources such as starches, sugars and cellulose;
• the use of physically milder conditions of temperature and pressure;

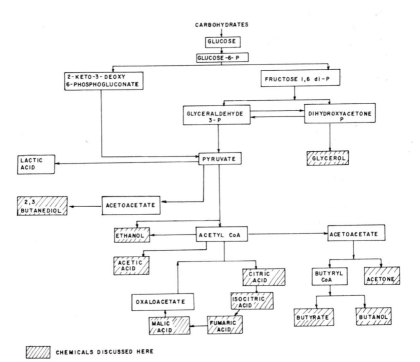

Figure 6-1. Basic pathway. Modified from Ref. 2.

- one-step production method where the need for intermediates separation and purification is bypassed;
- decreased pollution by the use of highly specific reactions offering finer control over products and byproducts.

Unfortunately such promises are balanced by:

- the cost and difficulty of separating useful products from a very dilute solution;
- the need for expansive cofactors;
- the difficulties associated with scale-up.

Table 6-1 summarizes the key chemicals produced by fermentation in the past and currently. The list is not very long. One of the reasons for this scarcity of commercial enzymatic reactions is that, unfortunately, much effort has gone into studying enzymes for their degradation properties and less attention has been given to their synthetic capability [8].

The purpose of this survey is to examine the optimistic and undocumented proposition that biotechnology will play a significant role in the growth, development and restructuring of the chemical industry. A systematic review of all branches of chemistry is not possible. We review in some detail aliphatic organic compounds, specialty chemicals, bulk commodity chemicals and alcohol and chemicals from biomass.

THE STRUCTURE OF THE INDUSTRY

Industrial chemistry is characterized by diversity and unity. Diversity is found in the 63,000 chemicals used in commerce. Unity is associated with the fact that of the 210 billion pounds of organic chemicals produced in the U.S., 99% are accounted by the top 100. Of these 100 major organics, 74% are produced from five primary feedstocks: ethylene; propylene; benzene; toluene; and xylene [2].

In 1981, industrial firms spent 1.3 billion on basic research or about 4% of the total industry-financed R&D expenditures. The investment in basic research by industry grew at an annual rate of 6.5% between 1975 and 1981. A large part of the increase in chemical research is associated with genetic engineering and other biotechnologies.

Unit Processes

The large number of chemical species and chemical reactions used in industrial processes make it difficult to understand this sector.

TABLE 6-1. Chemicals by Microbial Fermentation.

Compound	Structure	Microorganism	Carbon Source
Organic Acids			
Acetic acid	CH_3COOH	Acetobacter aceti	Ethanol
Citric acid	$HOO-C-(CH_2COOH)_2$ $\|$ OH	Aspergillus niger Candida lipolytica Candida guilliermondii	Sucrose n-alkane cellulose
Gluconic acid	$COOH$ $\|$ $(CHOH)_4$ $\|$ CH_2OH	Aspergillus niger	Glucose
Itaconic acid	$COOH$ $\|$ $C=H_2$ $\|$ CH_2COOH	Aspergillus terreus	Glucose
Lactic Acid	$COOH$ $\|$ $CHOH$ $\|$ CH_3	Lactobacillus delbrueckii	glucose

(continued)

TABLE 6-1. (continued).

Compound	Structure	Microorganism	Carbon Source
Malic acid	COOH | CHOH | CH₂COOH	Brevibacterium flavum	fumaric acid
Adipic acid	HOOC(CH₂)₄COOH	Pseudomonas sp.	alkane
Propionic acid	CH₃CH₂COOH	Propionibacterium shermanii	glucose
Tartaric acid	COOH | (CHOH)₂ | COOH	Gluconobacter suboxydans	glucose
Acrylic acid	CH₂=CH COOH	Lactobacillus bulgarius clostridium propionium	glucose
Fumaric acid	COOH | H—C C—H | COOH	Candida lipolytica	n-alkane
D-arabrorscorbic acid		penicillium notatum	glucose
L-alloisocitric acid		penicillium purporogenum	glucose

(continued)

73

TABLE 6-1. (continued).

Compound	Structure	Microorganism	Carbon Source
L-isocitric acid	COOH | H—C—OH | HOOC—C—H | C—H | COOH	Candida brumptii	glucose
2-ketogluconic acid	HOOCCO[CH(OH)]₃ CH₂OH	Pseudomonas fluoresrens	glucose
5-ketogluconic	COOH | C=O | (CHOH)₃ | CH₂OH	Gluconobacter suboxydans	glucose

α-ketogluconic acid	O H
	‖ |
	HOOC—C—C—(CHOH₂—CH₂OH)
	       |
	       H
		Candida hydrocarbofumarica	n-alkane

(continued)

TABLE 6-1. (continued).

Compound	Structure	Microorganism	Carbon Source
Kojic acid		Aspergillus oryzae	glucose
Pyruvic acid	O $\parallel$ $HOOC-C-CH_3$	Pseudomonas aeruginosa	glucose
Succinic acid	CH_2COOH $\mid$ CH_2-COOH	Bacterium succinicum	malic acid
Alcohols			
Ethanol	CH_3CH_2OH	Sacchadomyces cerevisiae Zymomonas mobilis	glucose
Butanol	$CH_3CH_2CH_2CH_2OH$	Clostridium autianticum	glucose
Isopropanol	$CH_3CH\ CH_3$ $\mid$ OH	Clostridium aurianticum	glucose
Others			
Acetone	O $\parallel$ CH_3-C-CH_3	Clostridium acetobutylicum	glucose
Ethylene glycol	$HOCH_2CH_2OH$	Saccharomyces cerevisiae Zymomonas mobilis	glucose

(continued)

TABLE 6-1. (continued).

Compound	Structure	Microorganism	Carbon Source
Glycerol	HOCH₂CHCH₂OH $\|$ OH	Saccharomyces cerevisiae	glucose
2,3 butane diol	CH₃CHOHCHOHCH₃	Bacillus polymyxa Aeromonas hydrophilia Bacillus subtilis Serratia marcessens	glucose
B Carotene		Mycobacterium smegmatis Blakeslea trispora	ammonium corn/soybean
methyl-ethyl ketone	CH₃COCH₂CH₃	Klebsiella pneumonia + chem. modif.	glucose
1,3 butadiene	CH₂=CH−CH=CH₂	Saccharomyces cerevisiae Zymomonas mobilis	glucose

It is possible to bring order by looking at unit processes rather than chemicals or reactions. A unit process is the traditional building block in manufacturing chemicals. For instance, the manufacture of toluene diisocyanate from toluene involves three unit processes: nitration of toluene to dinitrotoluene, hydrogenation of dinitrotoluene to diamino-toluene, and phosphogenation of diaminotoluene to toluene diiso-cyanate.

A comprehensive list of 39 commercially significant unit processes used in more than 5,000 plants to manufacture 263 principal chemicals in commerce has been complied. Twenty-three unit processes are con-sidered major (Table 6-2). Because they are used in many plants to pro-duce a number of different chemicals in large volume, 16 minor pro-cesses were also identified (Table 6-3) [9].

The major chemical industry unit processes have counterparts in the biological world. A few examples document this thesis.

Carbonylation

Carbonylation or the Oxo reaction, is the combination of an organic compound with carbon monoxide. It is a method of converting -olefins to aldehydes and/or alcohols containing one additional carbon atom.

The Monsanto carbonylation process for acetic acid manufacture reacts liquid methanol with gaseous carbon monoxide at 175 °C and 30 atm pressure in the presence of a soluble rhodium iodocarbonyl catalyst. The equation for the reaction is:

$$CH_3OH + CO \xrightarrow[175\,°C]{catalyst} CH_3COOH$$

The formation of acetic acid by *Acetobacter* is a practical example of enzymatic carbonylation.

$$C_2H_5OH + O_2 \xrightarrow{acetobacter} CH_3COOH + H_2O$$

Dehydrogenation

Dehydrogenation is the process by which a new chemical is formed by the removal of hydrogen from the feedstock compound. Aldehydes and ketones are prepared by the dehydrogenation of alcohols.

An example is the dehydrogenation of ethyl alcohol to acetaldehyde, as shown by the following equation:

TABLE 6-2. Major Unit Processes.

Process	Compounds
1. Alkylation	15
2. Amination by Ammonolysis	13
3. Ammoxidation	10
4. Carbonylation (oxo)	10
5. Condensation	55
6. Cracking (catalytic)	3
7. Dehydration	6
8. Dehydrogenation	15
9. Dehydrohalogenation	6
10. Esterification	24
11. Halogenation	54
12. Hydrodealkylation	3
13. Hydrogenation	27
14. Hydrohalogenation	7
15. Hydrolysis (hydration)	28
16. Nitration	12
17. Oxidation	47
18. Oxyhalogenation	5
19. Phosgenation	3
20. Polymerization	34
21. Pyrolysis	20
22. Reforming (steam)—Water Gas Reaction	1
23. Sulfonation	11
Total	410

Source: Ref. 9.

TABLE 6-3. Minor Unit Processes.

Process	Compounds
1. Acid Cleavage	2
2. Acid Rearrangement	3
3. Amination by Reduction	2
4. Beckmann Rearrangement	1
5. Benzidine Rearrangement	1
6. Cannizzaro Reaction	1
7. Carboxylation	5
8. Chlorohydrination	3
9. Electrohydrodimerization	1
10. Epoxidation	4
11. Hydroacetylation	1
12. Hydrocyanation	2
13. Isomerization	3
14. Oximation	1
15. Oxyacetylation	1
16. Ozonolysis	7
	38

Source: Ref. 9.

78

$$CH_3CH_2OH \xrightarrow[250-350\,°C]{Cu\ catalyst} CH_3\overset{\displaystyle O}{\overset{\|}{C}}H + H_2$$

An example of enzymatic dehydrogenation is the conversion of an alcohol to an aldehyde.

$$Ethanol + NAD \xrightarrow[Dehydrogenase]{alcohol} Acetaldehyde + NADH$$

Esterification

Esterification is the process by which an ester is formed. An ester is an organic compound derived from an organic acid and an alcohol by the exchange of the ionizable hydrogen atom of the acid for an organic radical. In transesterification, an ester reacts with an alcohol to form a different ester.

An example of esterification is the formation of ethyl acetate by the reaction of acetic acid and ethyl alcohol in the presence of a mineral acid catalyst, as shown by the following equation:

$$CH_3\overset{\displaystyle O}{\overset{\|}{C}}OH + C_2H_5OH \rightleftharpoons CH_3\overset{\displaystyle O}{\overset{\|}{C}}OC_2H_5 + H_2O$$

Using carboxyl esterase as a stereoselective catalyst and methyl propionate as a matrix ester, the following optically active alcohols and their propionic esters were produced on a preparative scale: 3-methoxy-1-butanol, 3-methyl-1-pentanol, 3,7-dimethyl-1-octanol and -citronellol [10].

$$CH_3CH_2\overset{\displaystyle O}{\overset{\|}{C}}OCH_3 + HOCH_2CH_2R \rightarrow$$

$$CH_3CH_2\overset{\displaystyle O}{\overset{\|}{C}}OCH_2CH_2R + CH_3OH$$

Halogenation

Halogenation is the process whereby a halogen is used to introduce one or more halogen atoms into an organic compound.

A process for the production of ethylene dichloride is the direct chlorination of ethylene in the presence of ferric chloride catalyst, as shown in the following equation:

$$CH{=}CH_2 \ + \ Cl_2 \xrightarrow[\text{135 C}]{\text{FeCl}} ClCH_2CH_2Cl$$

A large number of haloperoxidases are able to catalyze halogenation reactions (Cl^-, B^-, I^-). Among these are myeloperoxidase, chloroperoxidase, lactoperoxidase, bromoperoxidase, iodoperoxidase, horseradish, peroxidase.

An example of the formation of a dihalide derivative is as follows:

$$
\begin{array}{ccc}
\overset{\displaystyle OH}{\underset{\displaystyle |}{}} & \overset{\displaystyle OH}{\underset{\displaystyle |}{}} & \\
CH_2 - C = C - CH_2 & \xrightarrow[\text{chloroperoxidase}]{Cl^-/Br^-} & CH_2 - C = C - CH_2
\end{array}
$$

OH   Br Cl OH

Hydration

Hydration is the process in which water reacts with a compound without decomposition of the compound, forming a new compound containing both the hydrogen and hydroxyl groups. An example is the Veba-Chemie AG process for the production of isopropyl alcohol by the direct hydration of propylene with demineralized water, as shown by the following equation:

$$CH_3CH = CH_2 \ + \ H_2O \xrightarrow[\text{170–190 C}]{\text{catalyst}} (CH_3)_2CHOH$$

The hydration of areneoxide (benzene oxide) is a well known enzymatic reaction.

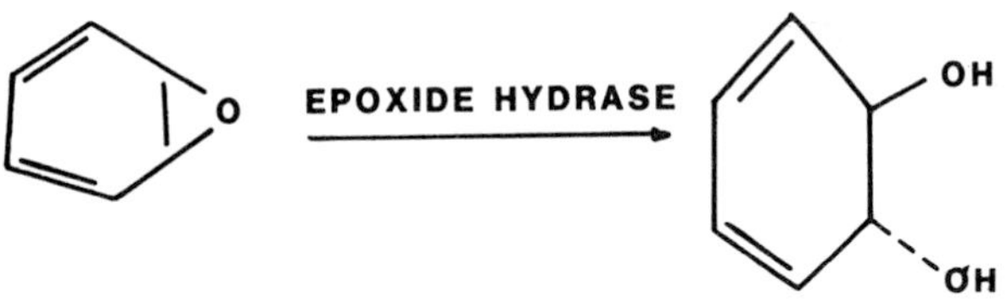

Oxidation

The unit process of oxidation of organic compounds generally means chemical reaction with oxygen to introduce one or more oxygen atoms into the compound, and/or to remove hydrogen atoms from the compound. The term "oxidation" has been broadened to include any reaction in which electrons are lost. Oxidation and reduction always occur simultaneously (redox reactions). The substance losing electrons is oxidized and the substance receiving electrons is reduced.

The oxidation process is used in the Aldehyd GmbH process for acetaldehyde production by the direct oxidation of ethylene. The process uses a catalyst solution of cupric chloride, which contains small quantities of palladium chloride. The reactions may be summarized as follows:

$$CH_2 == CH_2 + 2CuCl_2 + H_2O \xrightarrow{PdCl_2} CH_3CHO + 2CuCl + 2HCl$$

$$2CuCl + 2HCl + 1/2O_2 \rightarrow 2CuCl_2 + H_2O$$

Oxygenases are very common in biological systems. An example would be the oxidation of catechol via two pathways.

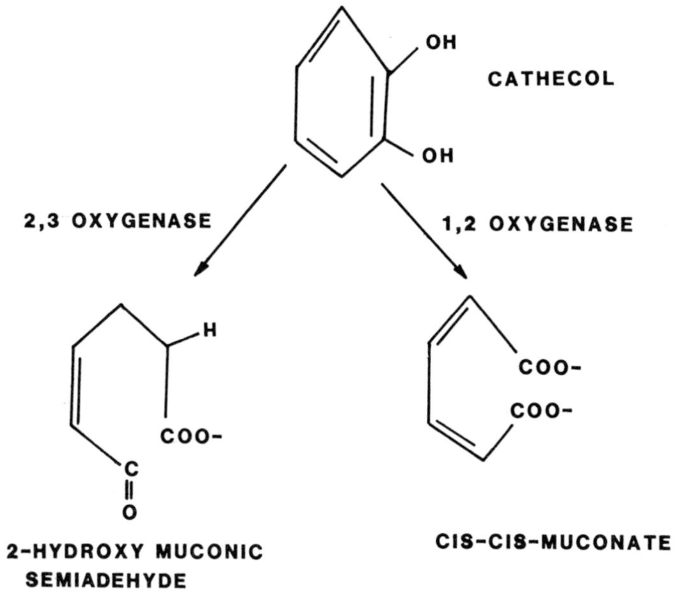

CATHECOL

2,3 OXYGENASE

1,2 OXYGENASE

2-HYDROXY MUCONIC SEMIADEHYDE

CIS-CIS-MUCONATE

Epoxidation

Epoxidation is the process by which an epoxide is formed. In epoxidation, an alkene reacts with a peracid, the pi bond of the alkene is broken, and a three-membraned cyclic ether called an epoxide, or oxirane, is formed. The generic equation for the reaction is:

$$\overset{\displaystyle\diagdown}{\underset{\displaystyle\diagup}{C}} = = \overset{\displaystyle\diagup}{\underset{\displaystyle\diagdown}{C} } + RC-O-OH \rightarrow \overset{\displaystyle O}{\underset{\displaystyle\diagup}{C}}\overset{\displaystyle\diagup\diagdown}{-----}\overset{\displaystyle\diagup}{\underset{\displaystyle\diagdown}{C}} + RC-OH$$

a peracid   an expoxide (oxirane)

The proposed Cetus process for the production of propylene oxide includes as epoxidation reaction

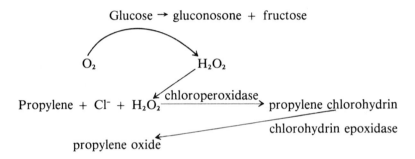

Glucose → gluconosone + fructose

$$O_2 \qquad H_2O_2$$

Propylene + Cl⁻ + H₂O₂ $\xrightarrow{\text{chloroperoxidase}}$ propylene chlorohydrin

$\qquad\qquad\qquad\qquad\qquad\qquad$ chlorohydrin epoxidase

propylene oxide

Isomerization

Isomerization is the process whereby an organic compound under the influence of heat and a catalyst is converted to another compound having different properties, by changing the arrangement of atoms in the molecule without changing the number of atoms.

The conversion of fructose 6- phosphate to glucose 6-phosphate is probably the best known example of an isomerization reaction by isomerase.

Polymerization

Polymerization is a chemical process in which a large number of relatively simple molecules combine to form a chain-like macromolecule. The reaction is usually carried out with a catalyst, often under high pressure.

Industrial polymerizations are performed by subjecting unsaturated or other reactive compounds to conditions that will bring about combination. Polymerizations generally can be divided into two types: (1) condensation polymerizations, in which polymers are formed by the elimination of small molecules, such as water; and (2) addition poly-merizations, in which saturation of one or more unsaturated bonds is effected. For the manufacture of nylon 66, an equimolar mixture of adipic acid and hexamethylenediamine is heated at 270 °C at 10 atm pressure. The equation for the reaction follows:

$$
\begin{array}{cc}
O & O \\
\| & \| \\
\end{array}
$$
$$
nHOC(CH_2)_4COH \ + \ nNH_2(CH_2)_6NH_2 \ \rightarrow
$$

$$
\begin{array}{cc}
O & O \\
\| & \| \\
\end{array}
$$
$$
\left.-NH\,C(CH_2)_4CNH(CH_2)_6-\right]_n \ + \ 2nH_2O
$$

Addition polymerization occurs in the manufacture of polyvinyl chloride from vinyl chloride. The polymerization can be carried out in a water suspension, which contains a soap as an emulsifier and a per-sulfate initiator. The equation for the reaction follows:

$$
nCH_2 = CH \rightarrow (-CH_2-CH-)_n
$$
$$
\qquad\quad |\qquad\qquad\quad \backslash
$$
$$
\qquad\quad Cl\qquad\qquad\quad Cl
$$

Polymerization is a very common process in biology. DNA is a poly-mer of four bases, proteins are polymers based on 20 amino acids. Cellulose, lignin and chitin are very abundant polymers.

As we can see from the few examples above, the chemical industry, in spite of its might and years of experience, has not invented much that was not already present in the humblest of bacteria.

ALIPHATIC ORGANIC COMPOUNDS

The production of chemicals in the U.S. requires the equivalent of 7-8% of the annual energy consumption, mostly in the form of petroleum and natural gas [11].

Of the 100 most important chemicals, only six are produced by fer-mentation routes and only in small quantity, with the exception of ethanol. Our world has many cyclical tendencies. A number of chemi-cals have been produced by biological means, to be abandoned with the appearance of abundant and cheap petroleum, only to return on the scene with signs of petroleum scarcity and high prices.

- Several fermentation processes were developed for glycerol production from molasses prior to 1960 [12].
- The aceteon/butanol fermentation process was highly successful and lasted in the U.S. from the early 1920's to the late 1950's.

A few examples given below document the technical feasibility of producing a wide range of aliphatic organic compounds by fermentation of inexpensive or well defined substrates.

Acrylic Acid

Because of its high market value (77¢/Kg) and potential high yield from glucose (0.8 g/g), acrylic acid is attractive as a product of an integrated biomass to ethanol process [13].

The oxidation of propionate to acrylic acid involves a minimum of four steps:

$$\text{propionate} \rightarrow \text{propionate} \rightarrow \text{propionyl CoA}$$

outside   inside
cells   cells

$$\rightarrow \text{acrylyl CoA} \rightarrow \text{acrylate}$$

When employing the anaerobic microorganism *Clostridium propionicum*, lactate by being converted to propionate stimulates acrylic acid production. Efforts have documented the effect of substrate concentration, cell mass, pH, ionic strength and oxygen tension. Much remains to be analyzed before a commercial process arises.

The Nitto Chemical Industries KK of Japan has announced an enzymatic hydrolysis process for the production of methacrylamide from metacrylonitrile.

$$\underset{\underset{CH_3}{|}}{CH_2} = C \equiv N + H_2O \xrightarrow{\text{enzyme}} \underset{\underset{CH_3}{|}}{CH_2} = C - \overset{\overset{O}{\|}}{C} - NH_2$$

This process operates at room temperature and has almost no undesirable byproducts [7].

Malic Acid

Malic acid used in the pharmaceutical industry and as a food additive is produced commercially by the enzymatic conversion of fumaric acid using immobilized cells of *Brevibacterium flavum*.

$$
\begin{array}{ccc}
\begin{array}{c}
\text{COOH} \\
| \\
\text{CH} \\
| \\
\text{HC} \\
| \\
\text{COOH} \\
\text{fumaric} \\
\text{acid}
\end{array}
& + \; H_2O \; \xrightarrow{\text{Fumarase}} &
\begin{array}{c}
\text{COOH} \\
| \\
\text{CH}_2 \\
| \\
\text{HCOOH} \\
| \\
\text{COOH} \\
\text{L-malic} \\
\text{acid}
\end{array}
\end{array}
$$

The malic world population is around 500 tons per year. Although malic acids can be extracted from the juices of fruits or by chemical synthesis; the only process in use is enzymatic [14].

Lactic Acid

Lactic acid can be produced by *Thermolactic bacterium* with cellulose as the only source of carbon [15]. *C. thermocellum* growing on cellulose will produce enough sugars to support the growth of *Thermolactic bacterium* and result in the accumulation of lactic acid. Typical conversion of 0.8–0.9g lactic acid per gram of glucose consumed was found. The technical feasibility of a commensalistic mixed culture has been demonstrated [13].

Acetic-Propionic-Butyric Acids

Adaptation and selection of strains to increase tolerance to acetate allows *Clostridium thermoaceticum* to produce interesting amount of acetic acid. Acetic acid concentrations in the range of 15–22 gm/liter are achieved at 59 °C in 32 hours [13,16,17].

A recent economic study demonstrated the economic advantages of the production of mixed acids (acetic and propionic acids) from grass. The conceptual plant is based on a 200 metric tons of orchard grass per day. The grass is first hydrolyzed to glucose and xylose which are fermented for 2.3 days by the action of *Propionibacterium acidipropioni*. A break even cost of 10.8¢/Kg (for a mixture of 14g/l propionic and 6g/l acetic acids) was computed, or $0.125/Kg for a 15% return on investment. This compares to the market price of acetic and propionic acids at $0.58/Kg and $.73/Kg respectively (1982 dollar value). Even when the cost of recovery of the two acids $0.139/Kg is added, the process appears to be economical [18].

Several organisms capable of growing on one-carbon compounds have been isolated. *Butyribacterium methylotrophicum* and *Eubac-*

terium limosom have been grown on methanol to produce volatile organic acids: acetic and butyric acids [19].

$$10CH_3OH + 2HCO_3^- \rightarrow 3C_3H_7COO^- + 10H_2O + H^+$$

Mutants of the parent strain can grow on CO alone producing acetate and a small amount of butyrate. These organisms appear to be very efficient in terms of cell growth and reduced end products (Ca 85%). The economics of the process were not analyzed.

Citric Acid

Most of the world citric acid is produced by fermentation of the fungus *Aspergillus niger*, 80-85% conversion of the initial substrate is not uncommon [20]. *Candida* yeasts are also used to produce citric acid by submerged fermentation of carbohydrates. Recently *Candida guilliermondii* has been investigated for the production of citric acid from cellulose [21]. Accumulation of citric and isocitric acid is associated with conditions of nitrogen starvation.

Investigations have shown that the direct conversion of cellulose to citric acid should be conducted in a two-stage process. The first stage being optimized for cell growth and hydrolysis; the second stage being optimized for citric acid synthesis. High density bioreactors can be used for large increases in productivity per reactor unit.

Acetone/Butanol

The Weizmann process for acetone/butanol production from the fermentation of *Clostridium* was commercialized as early as 1914 [22]. The basic simplified chemistry of the process is as follows [23]:

$$\text{Formic acid} \rightarrow CO_2 + H_2O$$

Glucose—
   └─Acetaldehyde —
                  ├─Ethan 1-ol 12%
                  ├─Acetic Acid → Acetoacetic → Acetone
                  │   Acid   30%
                  └─Aldol → Butyric Acid → Butan-1-ol 58%

The process gave good yields (6:3:1 ratio of butanol, acetone, ethanol) from a variety of feedstocks: cornmeal mash, starches from maize, rice and molasses.

By 1920 the chemical route to acetone (from propylene) and butanol (from ethylene) was already well established. Today acetone/butanol are produced by fermentation only in South Africa (10,000 tons of butanol/acetone per year).

Interest is growing in taking another look at using biomass for acetone/butanol production [22], in the light of advances in biology and engineering [13]. A recent economic study shows that the process would be attractive from corn and whey and sulfite liquors. The process still suffers of some fundamental problems that must be resolved.

Glycerol

Glycerol is recovered as a byproduct of soap and fatty acid production. In the U.S., glycerol is produced by the allyl chloride process, the acrolein process and the peracetic acid process [12].

Several fermentation processes for glycerol production from molasses were developed prior to 1960. Glycerol is still produced from anaerobic yeast fermentation of molasses by ICI in England [12].

An alternative process has been proposed making use of the halophilic green algae, *Dunaliella*. Under appropriate conditions, the algae can accumulate as much as 56% of its weight in glycerol. The advantages of the process are inexpensive substrate (carbon dioxide and sunlight) and the possibility of recovering -carotene and animal feed protein as byproducts.

The process requires large areas of inexpensive land, a sunny arid climate, the availability of cheap CO_2 (e.g., stack gases), and inexpensive labor.

A preliminary economic analysis has been completed of the algae process versus the allyl chloride process. The biological route came up better (75.2¢/Kg versus 88.8¢/Kg) although the capital costs for the biological route are very large. The situation would improve with increasing prices of petroleum.

Economics, the Great Common Denominator

Microbiology has had little impact on the production methods of basic chemicals and intermediates. This situation is likely to remain the same until important economic gains are achieved using the biological route [24]. An example makes this point forcefully. When acetic acid fermentation:

$$C_2H_5OH + O_2 \xrightarrow{\text{Acetobacter}} CH_3COOH + H_2O$$

was compared to the production of the same acid by the Reppe carbonylation process:

$$CH_3OH + CO \xrightarrow{\text{Cat. Co/I}_L} CH_3COOH$$

The fermentation process was found to be almost three times more expansive.

The end of the panic over oil scarcity and skyrocketing petroleum prices does not auger well for a large-scale biochemistry replacing the petro chemistry.

COMMODITY CHEMICALS

Is there a biotechnology future for bulk chemicals? Chemicals and allied products are a $169 billion business in 1982; some 10% of all manufacturing industries dollar volume [25]. It is, indeed, a large, well established business.

In 1982 the chemical industry used 2661 trillion Btu, 39% in the form of natural gas, 17.2% in the form of petroleum bases fuels; the remainder being electricity (29.7%), coal and coke (11.0%) and purchased steam (3.1%) [25]. The prospects of generally reducing energy use; and specifically the dependence on petroleum, are at the source of the renewed interest in fermentation and enzymatic reactions for large scale chemicals production.

Table 6-4 lists the 50 most important organic products in terms of 1982 production [25]. For each we indicate if a biological route to production was used in the past or is in current use; even if for partial production. We also indicate which of these organics has potential for biological production in the future, if the right conditions arise.

The prospects for producing large volumes of bulk commodity chemicals by microorganisms are not very good. A unique combination of factors would have to converge to insure such success: high priced petroleum, strong industrial demand, expanded export, and substantial economic advantages for the biological route.

SPECIALTY CHEMICALS

The trend toward specialties with their greater value added and higher pricing characteristics has not escaped the astute market specialists.

TABLE 6-4. Top Organic Chemicals.

Organic	1982 Production[1]	Biological Route[2]	Potential for Biotechnologies[3]
Acetic Acid	2,751	X	XXX
Acetone	1,757	X	XXX
Acrylonitrile	2,041		
Aniline	557		X
Benzene, mg	1,073		X
Bisphenol A	479		
1,3-butadiene	1,826		
Butanol	706	X	XXX
Caprolactam	797		
Carbon disulfide	n.a.		
Carbon tetrachloride	588		
Cumene	2,678		
Cyclohexane	1,272		
Diisodecyl phtalate	108		X
Dodecylbenzene	484		
Ethanol, synthetic	1,028	X	XXX
Ethanolamines	403		X
Ethylchloride	339		
Ethylbenzene	6,674		
Ethylene	24,683		
Ethylene dichloride	9,985		
Ethylene glycol	4,295		XX
Ethylene oxide	5,000		XX
2-ethyl hexanol	321		
Formaldehyde, 37%	4,691		X
Isopropyl alcohol	1,310		X
Maleic anhydride	259		
Methanol, synthetic	7,265		X
Methyl chloride	370		
Methylethyl ketone	462		X
Methyl chloroform	586		
Methylene chloride	524		
Perchloroethylene	585		
Phenol, synthetic	2,136		XX
Phthalic anhydride	691		X
Propylene	12,290		X
Propylene glycol	403		XX
Propylene oxide	n.a.		XX
Styrene, monomer	5,298		
Terephthalic acid, dimethyl ester	4,974		
Toluene, mg	1,057		
Vinyl acetate	1,876		
Vinyl chloride	6,495		
o-xylene	799		
p-xylene	2,926		

[1]In millions of pounds unless otherwise noted.
[2]Produced by biological route now or in the past.
[3]XXX = highly likely; XX = likely; X = possible.
Source: Mod. from Ref. 15.

A mad rush, if not a scrambling, is on toward specialty chemicals. With a 10.1% average annual growth over the last five years, they represent a challenging target [26]. In 1982, the specialty business totaled $40 billion. The specialty market is expected to grow to $60 billion by 1990 (Table 6-5).

Everything is not rosy. Individual specialty chemicals are produced in small quantities under intense competition. These conditions of high value added and intense competition are fertile grounds for innova-

TABLE 6-5. The Shape of Specialty Markets in 1990.

	U.S. Sales* Millions of dollars	
Segment	1982	1990
Oil Fields	$5,220	$9,195
Agriculture	5,300	6,715
Electronics	2,240	6,075
Industrial coatings	3,900	4,940
Specialty lubricants	3,200	3,615
Industrial and institutional cleaners	2,800	3,550
Specialty polymers	1,675	3,340
Diagnostics	1,400	3,000
Adhesives and sealants	1,500	2,600
Plastic additives	1,575	2,325
Lubricant additives	1,500	1,900
Food Additives	1,200	1,640
Photography	950	1,630
Catalysts	1,125	1,615
Water management	900	1,315
Textiles	750	1,025
Metal finishing	550	700
Biocides	500	685
Cosmetics	510	645
Specialty surfactants	400	640
Rubber	450	615
Reagents	350	515
Explosives	400	505
Paper	330	450
Refineries	250	370
Paint and coating additives	275	350
Mining	235	300
Fuel additives	200	275
Printing ink	165	210
Foundries	130	165
Total	$39,980	$60,905

*Constant 1982 dollars
Source: Ref. 26.

tions, including biotechnologies. Biotechnologies have already made great strides in certain submarkets such as diagnostics, pesticides and water treatment. They are poised to enter the oil fields, mining and agriculture sectors.

It is hard today to find a chemical company without some involvement in biotechnology, either through in-house research, contract research, or equity in a biotechnology firm. The well established companies are chasing every lead now while realizing that impact on sales and earnings is at least 15 years away, in most cases.

The health and environment concerns of the 1970's and the oil price shock of 1973-1974 have had important impacts on research and development, fostering defensive research to the detriment of new product innovations. The 1980's are heralding a return to fundamental research. By 1981, chemical companies had earmarked $3.2 billion of research funds to product innovation. In spite of this investment, new products represent only 20% of industry profit [27].

The growing interest on less dependence on commodity and more dynamism is propelling essentially all chemical companies to enter the specialty field.

The market oriented biotechnologist will pay attention to trends in the specialty chemicals sector.

- The replacement of hydrogen peroxide for chlorine oxide in the pulp and paper sector [28].
- Convenience food and extended shelf life demand chemical additives [29].
- The need to extract every possible drop of oil from established producer wells foster enhanced oil recovery [30,31].
- A society demanding sweetness without the calories.
- Vitamins are a dear product in a health conscious society.
- The growing family of uses for amino acids.
- Novel detergent formulae [32] with a rebirth for enzymes.
- Perfumers copying nature with pheromone-based fragrences [33].
- Organics leading the way in corrosion inhibitors [34].
- Water management chemicals need an injection of aggressive science and technology [35].
- Adhesives are looking for new applications and innovations [36].

Specialty chemical experts must recognize:

- An older and more educated consumer
- A shortened life cycle for new products
- Concern over the quality of the environment
- Interest in energy economical processes

- The need for extensive technical expertise
- The support of products with continuing services
- The regulatory burden associated with specialty chemicals
- The need for expensive and continued research and development

Some of the major areas where biotechnology can impact the specialty chemicals market include:

- amino acids
- sweeteners without calories
- vitamins
- polysaccharides
- dyes
- enzymes

CHEMICALS FROM BIOMASS

Cellulose, lignin and chitin are the most important forms of biomass, representing a virtually inexhaustive, self-renewing source of raw material. The basic component of cell walls is cellulose. Cellulose is made up of long chains of glucose molecules, a six-carbon sugar, joined by a 1,4-glucoside bond [37]. The chains fit together over part of their lengths to form a crystalline structure that gives the plant cell wall their strength and rigidity. If the cellulose molecules are hydrolyzed by acids or enzymes to glucose, the sugar can provide the substrate for many fermentation processes or can be chemically converted to ethylene glycol, sorbitol or surfactants.

Associated with the cellulose in the cell walls is hemicellulose. This is a lower molecular weight amorphous polymer made up of branched and linear chains of various sugars. In softwoods, about 20 percent of the dry weight is hemicellulose, made up largely of mannose and xylose. In hardwoods, about 30 percent of the dry weight is hemicellulose, made up largely of xylose. The hemicellulose is more readily hydrolyzed than is cellulose [38].

Plant cells, made up largely of cellulose and hemicellulose, are coated with and bound together by lignin. Lignin is constructed of substituted phenylpropyl units linked to form a 3-dimensional polymer. The specific substituents and linkages vary with the plant species. Lignin makes up about 20–24% of hardwoods and 28% of softwoods. Lignin is soluble in alkaline solutions, and oxygenated organic solvents such as ethanol, acetone, phenol, n-butanol, and amines [38].

Hardwood is typically 52% carbon, 41% oxygen, 6% hydrogen, and less than 1% ash, along with small amounts of nitrogen and traces of sulfur. This contrasts with the traditional chemical feedstocks. Natural gas is over 75% carbon with trace amounts of oxygen. Petroleums range from 83–92% carbon with very little oxygen. This difference in level of carbon and more importantly in oxygen content has two major implications for chemicals from biomass. The basic unit processes for biomass-based chemicals will tend to be reductive rather than the oxidative reactions widely used in petrochemistry today. The more oxygen that is eliminated to build the final product, the greater the penalty in feedstocks cost that will be paid for the chemical from biomass. For this reason, final products with a relatively high oxygen content are more likely to be competitive with petrochemicals [38].

There are two basic approaches to the conversion of wood to chemicals. First, the major components of wood are separated and converted into various chemicals which preserve the basic structure of the lignocellulose feedstocks. In the second approach, the wood is gasified to carbon oxides and hydrogen.

The separation of wood into its chemical components is a difficult task. These components are intricately bonded together into a structure that resists biological degradation. Most approaches use some form of pre-treatment to expose the components to attack. The method of grinding or milling is energy-intensive because of the fibrous structure of wood, however, this approach has been used successfully on municipal solid waste [38].

The steam-explosion process breaks apart the fibers and expose the cellulose and hemicellulose to hydrolysis. These methods of pre-treatment achieve a partial hydrolysis of the hemicellulose and leave a high-quality, reactive lignin. Some workers have taken this pre-treatment a step further, and achieved a high degree of autohydrolysis of both the hemicellulose and cellulose. They use extruder-type devices in which the feedstock is subjected to elevated temperature and pressure along with dilute sulfuric acid, followed by rapid decompression. Recently a form of freeze-explosion using ammonia has been announced as a pre-treatment [39]. Other alternatives include gamma irradiation and treatment with hydrogen fluoride or nitric acid [38].

A somewhat different approach to pre-treatment involves solvent delignification which produces a highly reactive lignin and leaves the cellulose and hemicellulose exposed for hydrolysis. Other approaches use a mild alkali solvent that also removes some of the hemicellulose; or ethanol and phenol extraction solvents, respectively to remove lignin and hemicellulose and leaves behind a high quality cellulose that can be used for its fiber value or subjected to hydrolysis [38].

Once the cellulose and hemicellulose have been exposed, there are two options for conversion to sugars—acid or enzymatic hydrolysis. Acid hydrolysis is a two-step process. The hemicellulose is hydrolyzed under initial mild conditions to 5-carbon sugars with some 6-carbon sugars. Then the cellulose is subjected to a stronger acid hydrolysis to yield glucose. The sugars produced by acid hydrolysis are then available for fermentation.

There are a number of variations in the enzymatic hydrolysis option. One process performs both the hydrolysis (saccharification) and the fermentation in a single-step by using a combination of organisms: *Trichoderma reesei* and mutant strains of *Candida brassicae*. Other processes separate the saccharification and the fermentation step because of the difficulty of finding organisms that will perform these two functions optimally at the same reaction conditions. Most fermentations, however, currently use only the 6-carbon sugars. Effort has also been directed toward the identification and development of organisms that will ferment 5-carbon sugars to ethanol. Prime candidates are *Candida* and *Pachysolens* [38].

In general, the enzymatic processes for hydrolysis are lagging the chemical process in commercial readiness. A number of the laboratory enzymatic hydrolysis processes work well on pure cellulose or particular feedstocks, but not on the complex and varied feedstocks that would be used under industrial conditions.

In the past, the enzymatic route has not progressed as rapidly as the chemical (acid hydrolysis) route. Recent progress in enzymology and fermentation will change this picture dramatically.

- The ability of *Pachysolen tannophilus* to convert pentoses (xylose) to ethanol and carbon dioxide (NRC Canada, USDA).
- The discovery that *Cyathus stercoreus* can break down lignin (USDA).
- The well demonstrated capability of *Trichoderma reesei* and *T. viridex* (Cleveland State U.) to break down cellulose.
- The observation that *Clostridium thermocellum* and *C. thermosaccharolyticum* can break down starches and ferment the sugar simultaneously (MIT).
- Progresses made in butanol fermentation using *Clostrium acatobutylicum* (Kansas State) and in ethanol production using *Zymomonas mobilis* (University of Queenland, Australia).
- New strains of *Candida* to ferment both glucose and xylose substrates (Purdue University).

The enzymatic conversion of cellulose waste to glucose is due to the action of cellulase from mutant fungus strains. The crude glucose is then used in a microbial fermentation process to produce alcohols, chemical feedstocks and single cell proteins.

Methane can be produced in anaerobic digester from manure and other biological waste material. Algae can produce liquid hydrocarbons by reacting microscopal green plants with inexpensive hydrogen.

Ethanol, furfural, phenol, acetic acid, n-butanol, maleic anhydride, lignosulfonates, etc., are all possible products derived from bio-refineries. Recombinant DNA is being used to engineer better micro-organisms.

The second alternative for the conversion of biomass to chemicals is gasification and synthesis. In this approach, the problems of separation of wood components is avoided by the partial oxidation of the biomass to synthesis gas, a mixture of carbon monoxide and hydrogen. From these simple but reactive molecules, more complex chemicals are built by the proper choices of temperature, pressure, catalyst, and hydrogen/carbon monoxide ratio [38].

The chemistry of carbon monoxide, frequently called C_1 chemistry, has been developing rapidly in recent years, driven by the long-term prospect of conversion to gasified coal as the basic feedstock. C_1 chemistry was used to produce synthetic gasoline in Germany during World War II. This Fischer-Tropsch catalytic synthesis was largely dropped as inexpensive natural gas and then Near Eastern petroleum became available. Development has continued at the Sasol I, II and III facilities in South Africa where low-grade coal is converted to liquid propane gas (LPG), ethylene, alcohols, gasoline and diesel fuel. The original Fischer-Tropsch reactions were highly unspecific, producing over 100 products in mixture. Research is now being directed to specific catalysts, and targets of interest are the production of C_2-C_4 hydrocarbons and the production of branched hydrocarbons for aniti-knock properties and for lubricating oils [38].

The direct conversion from synthesis gas that is attracting the most commercial interest is methanol. A number of fuels, fuel additives and chemicals can be derived from methanol. These chemicals include for-maldehyde, acetic acid and methyl chloride and, with commercializa-tion of new routes, ethylene glycol, ethylene and propylene.

Although ethylene can be produced from biomass either by a Fischer-Tropsch process or by the dehydration of ethanol, it is not likely to make economic sense in the United States at this time, to produce a non-oxygenated petrochemical feedstock from biomass.

Ammonia is produced from the hydrogen derived from synthesis gas. Carbon dioxide is a by-product. Natural gas is the preferred feedstock because it produces a synthesis gas rich in hydrogen. Biomass is a possi-ble feedstock but would not be ideal for industrial scale facilities. The output of a large biomass facility would be about 500 tons of ammonia per day. The industrial facilities of this size that are based on natural gas have been shown to be too small to be competitive. The develop-ment of modularized farm scale ammonia plants, however, might make economic sense in agricultural areas rich in biomass residues [38].

The two major technical issues in the gasification-synthesis route to chemicals from biomass are selective, long-life catalysts and feedstocks variability demanding new gasifier designs.

Lignin can be the starting material for many industrial chemicals. Phenol derivatives and hydrocarbons by hydrogenation, phenol derivatives and cathecols by hydrolysis, vanilin by oxidation and organic sulfur compounds. Lignin obviously could also be used in polymeric forms for materials in which its function would be similar to its role in the native environment: as thermosetting resins, as components in polymers, as antioxidants, rubber reinforcements, dispersants and emulsion stabilizers [40].

Twenty-two million tons per year of lignin are generated by the U.S. pulp and paper industry and is used as a low cost boiler fuel [41].

T. fermentaus accumulates low molecular weight phenolic products as a result of lignin depolymerization. Eugenol, cinnanil acid, cinnamaldehyde, guaiacol, ferulic acid, vanillin, vanillic acid, and protocatechoic acid have been detected [42].

Chitisan is derived from chitin by deacetylation. Because of its functional properties, material characteristics and abundance, it has great, as yet unexploited, industrial potential [43–45]. A variety of uses have been proposed: adhesive, chelating agent, coagulant, drug carrier, membrane, paper and textile additives, photographic products, surgical adjuncts, structural matrix, textile finishers [43].

Chitin is a polymer of n-acetyl-glucosamine. It is a close relative of cellulose. Chitin is one of the most widely distributed polymers. The global industrial production is estimated at 150,000 tons per year. The biological production, as part of marine custracean shell, is immense.

A variety of species are being studied as a source of crude oil. The eukaryotic alga *Botryococcus braunii* is such an organism. Crude oil content may reach 50% of dry weight. The crude oil contains a lipid and an hydrocarbon fraction. The hydrocarbons are C_{27} to C_{31} linear di-and tri-alpha-olefins. These are valuable feedstocks that could be cracked to chemical feedstocks. The protein content of the cell may reach as high as 30%.

CHEMICALS FROM THE DESERT AND THE SEA

To many, space is the only remaining frontier. To the biochemist, the sea and the desert life are largely unknown.

Seventy percent of the earth is covered by oceans. Eighty percent of the total photosynthetic carbon fixation occurs in the open ocean of the continental surface. Thirty percent of the earth is covered by desert regions, including the arctic.

In principle, these vast expanses should be ideal for producing chemicals of interest to man. In practice, a number of drugs of actual and potential physiological and pharmacological action have been isolated and tested.

The only chemicals produced from these sources on a large scale are algal gums (agar, carrageenan, algin). Beta-carotene and glycerol are also produced from algae. One company, Ocean Genetics, is attempting to remedy the situation.

Chlorine and bromine are abundant in sea waters. The ratio of Cl^-/ Br^- is 500 (500 mM Cl^-/1 mM Br^1). It is not surprising that marine organisms store a wide variety and diversity of clorinated and brominated organic compounds. Because of their diversity, marine organisms produce some banal and some extraordinary compounds. Some of the most interesting compounds are heterogeneous dihalide derivatives [47].

CONCLUSION

Projection of $522 million/year by 1990 and $7.2 billion/year by 2000, have been made for the value of industrial chemicals produced by biotechnologists [48]. Only a small portion of this potential is likely to be realized.

Important success should occur in the biotechnology of drugs (e.g., aspirin), alphatic organic chemicals (e.g., acetic acid, ethanol), and specialty chemicals (e.g., amino acids, vitamins, polysaccharides). Few commodity chemicals will successfully compete with well established chemical processes.

A number of recent announcements are indicative of the vitality of the field:

- The Cetus production of propylene oxide by a two-step enzymatic process [49]. The following pathway is involved.

$$\text{D-Glucose} + O_2 \xrightarrow{\text{Pyranose-2 Oxidase}} H_2O_2 + \text{D-Gluconosone} \xrightarrow{H_2} \text{Fructose}$$

$$\text{Propylene} + Cl^- + H_2O_2 \xrightarrow{\text{Haloperoxidase}} \text{Propylene Chlorohydrin}$$
$$\searrow \text{Halohydrin epoxidase}$$
$$\text{Propylene oxide} + H^+ + Cl^-$$

This process has been placed on the back burner by Cetus.

- The production of long chain monohydric alcohols and acids by Chem. Systems.
- Production of dibasic acids and fragrance compounds by Synergen.
- The production of indigo and related dyes by Amgen. An *E. coli* strain containing the *Pseudomonas putida* gene for the conversion of naphthalene to a variety of compounds. The process involves the conversion of tryptophane to indole (by a tryptophanase), the oxydation of indole by naphthalene dioxygenase to indoxyl with subsequent dimerisation to indigo [50].
- The interest by Biochem./Hull, Ltd. to make organophosphorous compounds (total U.S. production over \$1 billion) widely used in agricultural chemicals, cosmetics, flame retardant, food products, lubricants, pharmeceuticals, plastic additives, plasticizers and surfactants. A few organophosphorous chemicals, guanosine monophosphate and fructose diphosphate, are currently made via fermentation [51].
- Genetic Internationals has contracted Cranfield Polytechnic (UK) for processes to make aromatic industrial chemicals by biotechnology.
- The bacterium, *Alcagines eutrophus* feeding on glucose, is being used in a process (ICI) to produce the polymer polyhydroxy butyrate ($[^-CH(CH_3)CH_2COO^-]n$). The polymer has high tensile strength and can be molded into hard consumer items [52,53].
- The production of 4,4'-dihydroxybiphenyl by strains of *Absioia pseudocylindrospura* 4,'4-dihydroxybiphenyl is one of the monomers used in the synthesis of union carbide sulfonebiphenol engineering polymer Radel [54].
- A fermentation method for producing the deicer calcium magnesium acetate [55].
- The study into the direct production of ethylene by mutant strains of the fungus *Penicillum digitatum* [56].
- An enzymatic route for the production of hydrazine [57].

These few examples document the vitality of the field and the many directions being pursued by industry.

REFERENCES

1. Perlman, D., "Fermentation Industries . . . Quovadis?" *ChemTech*, 430–443 (July 1977).

2. Ng, T. K., R. M. Busche, C. C. McDonald, and R. W. F. Hardy, "Production of Feedstock Chemicals," *Science, 219*, 733–740 (1983).

3. Zaborsky, O. R., "Enzymatic Production of Chemicals," in *Chemrawn I.* Pergammon Press (1978).

4. Bassham, J. A., "Photosynthesis and Biosynthetic Pathways to Chemicals," in *Chemrawn I.* Pergammon Press (1978).

5. Wright, P., "Time for Bug Valley," *New Scientist,* 27–29 (5 July 1979).

6. Eveleigh, D. E., "The Microbial Production of Industrial Chemicals," *Sci. Am., 245* (3), 155–178 (1981).

7. Mason, E. O., "Potential of Genetic Engineering and Biotechnology in Chemicals and Energy," in *Genetic Engineering and the Engineer,* National Academy Press, Washington, D.C. (1982).

8. National Academy of Sciences, "Degradation of Synthetic Organic Molecules in the Biosphere," NAS, Wash. D.C. (1972).

9. Herrick, E. C., J. A. King, R. P. Ouellette, and P. N. Cheremisinoff. *Unit Processes Series, Organic Chemical Industries,* Vol. 1, Ann Arbor Science Publ., Inc., Ann Arbor, MI (1977).

10. Cambou, B. and A. M. Klibanov, "Preparative Production of Optically Active Esters and Alcohols Using Esterase-catalyzed Streospecific Transesterification in Organic Media," MIT Report 6-27-83 (1983).

11. Culberson, D. L. and T. L. Donaldson, "Chemicals from Biomass: A Systems Analysis," *Biotech. & Bioeng. Symp., 12,* 291–296 (1982).

12. Chen, B. J. and C. H. Chi, "Process Development and Evaluation for Algal Glycerol Production," *Biotech. and Bioeng., 23,* 1267–1287 (1981).

13. Wang, D. I., C. L. Cooney, A. L. Demain, R. F. Gomez, and A. J. Sinskey, "Degradation of Cellulose Biomass and Its Subsequent Utilization for the Production of Chemical Feedstocks," U.S. Dept. of Energy, COO-418-6 (1978).

14. Chibata, I., T. Tosa, and I. Taknta, "Continuous Production of L-malic Acid by Immobilized Cells," *Trends in Biotechnology, 1* (1), 9–11 (1983).

15. Fields, M. L., A. M. Hamad, and D. K. Smith, "Natural Lactic Acid Fermentation of Cornmeal," *J. Food Science, 46,* 900–902 (1981).

16. Tong, G., "Fermentation Routes . . . C_3 and C_4," *Chemicals,* 70–74 (April 1978).

17. Sanderson, J. E., D. L. Wise, and P. C. Augenstein, "Organic Chemicals and Liquid Fuels from Algae Biomass," *Biotechnol. Bioeng. Symp., 8,* 131–151 (1979).

18. Clausen, E. C., R. B. Shah, G. Najafpour, and J. L. Gaddy, "Production of Organic Acids from Biomass by Acid Hydrolysis and Fermentation," *Biotech. & Bioeng. Symp., 12,* 67–72 (1982).

19. Datta, R., "Acidogenic Bioconversion of C_1 Compounds," *Biotechnology Bioeng. Symp., 12,* 177–182 (1982).

20. Kiel, H., R. Gurvin, and Y. Henis, "Citric Acid Fermentation by *Asperoclius niger* on Low-Sugar Concentrations and Cotton Waste," *Appl. & Env. Microbiol., 42* (1), 1–4 (1981).

21. Asendo, J. A., J. Szuhay, and D. Chio, "Growth and Citric-acid Production by *Candida guilliramondii* Using a Cellulose Substrate," *Biotechnology and Bioengineering Symp., 12,* 111–120 (1982).

22. Volesky, B., A. Mulchandani, and J. Williams, "Biochemical Production of Industrial Solvents (Acetone-Butanol-Ethanol) from Renewable Resources," in *Biochemical Engineering II,* A. Constantinides, W. R. Vieth, and K. Venkatasubramian, eds., The New York Academy of Sciences, NY (1981).

23. Gibbs, D. F., "The Rise and Fall (. . . and Rise?) of Acetone/Butanol Fermentations," *Trends of Biotechnology, 1* (1), 12–15 (1983).

24. Pape, M., "The Competition Between Microbial and Chemical Processes for the Manufacture of Basic Chemicals and Intermediates," in *Microbial Energy Conversion*, H. G. Schlegel and J. Branla, eds., Pergammon Press, Oxford (1976).

25. "Facts and Figures for the Chemical Industry," *CEN*, 27–67 (June 1983).

26. "The Urgent Rush to Specialty Markets," *Chemical Week*, 40–52 (Oct. 21, 1983).

27. "The All-Out Search for New Products That Pay," *Chemical Week*, 46–52 (Nov. 15, 1983).

28. "The Revival's on for Chemicals in Pulp and Paper," *Chemical Week*, 10–14 (Nov. 23, 1983).

29. "Food-Additives Market Will Double in 1980s," *Chemical Week*, 55–56 (Feb. 20, 1983).

30. "Oil Field Chemicals Still Awaiting Recovery," *C&EN*, 15–16 (Oct. 31, 1983).

31. Heaney, C. K., "Oil Field Chemicals: RIP for Ever?" *Chemical Business*, 35–39 (Nov. 14, 1983).

32. "Chelates Future: It'll Come Out in the Wash," *Chemical Business*, 31–39 (May 2, 1983).

33. "Perfumers Get Down to Basics," *Chem. Mrkt. Rept.*, 6 (March 17, 1983).

34. "Organics Lead the Way in Corrosion Inhibitors," *Chemical Marketing Reporter*, 38 (Feb. 7, 1983).

35. Brown, A. S., "Ebbtide for Water Management Chemicals," *Chemical Business*, 17–23 (Aug. 23, 1983).

36. "For Adhesives Makers There's Plenty of Action," *Chemical Week*, 14–15 (Oct. 19, 1983).

37. Kirk-Othmer, in *Encyclopedia of Chemical Technology*, 3rd edition, John Wiley, New York (1979).

38. Johnson, R. C., C. G. Miller, M. B. Neuworth, and A. Talib, *Chemicals from Wood: Policy Implications of Federal Subsidy*, Vol. 1, The MITRE Corp., MTR 83W9-01 (1983).

39. Dale, B. E. and M. J. Moreira, "A Freeze-Explosion Technique for Increasing Cellulose Hydrolysis," Fourth Symposium on Biotechnology in Energy Production and Conservation, Gatlinsburg, TN (May 11, 1982).

40. Kringstad, K., "The Challenge of Lignin," *Chemran I*, Pergammon Press (1978).

41. Graff, G. M., "High-Grade Lignin Schemes Edge Closer to Reality," *Chem. Eng.*, 25–27 (Dec. 27, 1982).

42. Cooney, C. L., A. L. Demain, A. J. Sinskey, and D. L. C. Wang, "Degradation of Lignocellulosic Biomass and Its Subsequent Utilization for the Production of Liquid Fuels," MIT, Report 6-22-83 (1983).

43. Rha, C., "Chitosan as a Biomaterial," MIT, Report 9-64-83D (1983).

44. Rodriquez-Sanchez, D. and C. Rha, "Chitosan Globules," MIT, Report 9-64-83E (1983).

45. The MIT Report, "Chitin: A Versatile Material from Nature," MIT (1983).

46. Pariser, R., "Overview of Chitin Research," MIT, Report 9-64-83A (1983).

47. Neidleman, S. L. and J. Geigert, "The Enzymatic Synthesis of Heterogeneous Dihalide Derivatives: A Unique Biocatalytic Discovery," *Trends in Biotechnology, 1* (1), 20–25 (1983).

48. "What Applied Genetics Might Do in Chemicals," *Chemical Week*, 41 (March 4, 1981).

49. Parkinson, G., "Enzyme Path to Products Is Traced at Meeting," *Chemical Engineering,* 37–39 (July 15, 1980).

50. Ensley, B. D., B. J. Ratzkin, T. D. Osslund, M. J. Simon, L. P. Wackett, and D. T. Gibson, "Expression of Naphthalene Oxidation Genes in *Escherichia coli* Results in the Biosynthesis of Indigo," *Science, 222,* 167–169 (1983).

51. "Making Organophosphorus Compounds. Is This Another Biotech Possibility," *Biomass Digest, 9* (4) (1982).

52. Mannon, J. H., "British Route to Polymer Hinges on Bacteria," *Chem. Eng.,* 41 (May 4, 1981).

53. "ICI Launches 'Biocol' to Commercialize its Microbe-Made Plastics," *Newswatch, 5* (June 20, 1983).

54. Schwartz, R. D., A. L. Williams, and D. B. Hutchinson, "Microbial Degradation of 4,4'-dihydroxy Biphenyl Hydroxylation by Fungi," *Natl. Env. Microbiol., 39* (4), 702–708 (1980).

55. "Road Deicer Researchers Take the Genetic Route," *Chem. Eng.,* 27–28 (May 2, 1983).

56. "New Route to Ethylene: Project to Try Fungal Fermentation," *Biomass Digest* (June 8, 1982).

57. "Enzymatic Route to Hydrazine," *Chemical Week,* 44 (Oct. 2, 1982).

7

Biotechnology and the Pharmaceutical Industry

FIRST WORD   In the beginning God created heaven and the earth. And the earth was without form and void; and darkness was upon the face of the deep.

GENESIS

There was a time when the massive Rocky Mountains were only a whispered rumor. There was a time when life could be explained only by the presence of a vital element. In both cases, curiosity and science have cleared the mist only to discover greater complexities. Today, a curiosity so vast has taken hold of man. It has become a love and a priesthood—it is called technology. Technology is usually equated with microelectronics and robotics. Now the hardware and the software of life have joined the high technology revolution. The wilderness and biology are again frontiers. Most important discoveries are made at frontiers or at interphases where old beliefs and new knowledge collide.

Nowhere, more than in the biotechnologist's laboratory, is the celebration of life put to the test. The scientific discoveries have been rewarding, the financial and societal benefits are promising.

Biotechnology was born in universities: in the medical faculty, the biology department and the pharmacy school. Today it is spreading to other units of science: engineering, chemistry, and computer sciences. Because of this origin and because it is a fiscally healthy sector, pharmacy is more often than not a first market for new ideas in biotechnology. The pharmaceutical sector is indeed vast. Only a few areas where biotechnology is expanding rapidly will be reviewed: diagnostic tests using monoclonal antibodies and DNA probes; vaccines, antibiotics, hormones and growth factors, and therapeutic programs.

The first word is one of ebullient hope, unbounded possibilities, joyous discoveries, exquisite variety and creative diversity.

103

MONOCLONAL ANTIBODIES

Antibodies are protein produced in our body as a defense against invasion of bacteria, viruses and other foreign matter. The human body may make as many as a hundred million antibody molecules, each recognizing a different antigen [1].

Traditionally, antibody (polyclonal antisera) have been produced in animals and purified from their blood. This technique suffers from severe limitations: batch to batch variation, limit on the quantity produced, and multiple specificities of the antisera. Monoclonal antibodies produced by single clones of antibody-producing cells can be extracted with great purity and in unlimited quantities.

Production

The production of monoclonal (pure clones) antibody is rather simple. An antigen (a foreign substance to an organism) of interest is injected into a mouse. A few days later the mouse's spleen is removed. It contains large amounts of white cells producing antibodies to the antigen injected. These cells are mixed with fast dividing cancer cells—myelomas and a chemical, polyethylene glycol (to effect fusion between the two kinds of cells). The result is an hybridoma. The fusion of the antibody-producing cells with the fast dividing cancer cells provides a product retaining both capabilities: virtually dividing forever and producing an endless supply of pure antibodies. The hybridoma is usually kept alive in a mouse, which is tapped at regular intervals, to retrieve material from which the antibodies are separated.

Many refinements are taking place in the technology for producing monoclonal antibodies (MAB). Damon recently announced hybridomas grown in microcapsules yielding concentration 30 to 100 times higher than those achieved in conventional tissue culture systems. At the University of Pennsylvania a part of gene or genes is inserted into antibody producing cells, immortalizing the cell line. Celltech developed an airlift fermenter for growing hybridoma in large quantities and almost continuously [2]. A successful in vitro technique for producing MAB has been developed at the General Hospital in Providence, RI [3].

It is possible to produce MAB against any specific antigen. The specificity, speed, and sensitivity of the antigen antibody reaction make it an ideal detector for complex molecules present in small quantity in a mixture of other chemical species. MAB can be engineered for detecting infectious agents, viruses, cell surface markers, hormones, and chemicals in general.

Monoclonal antibodies are now available to precisely identify lymphocytes and accurately quantify subtypes of T cells (e.g., helper, supresser), and the immunoglobin chains secreted by β-lymphocytes and those expressed on their surface.

MAB specifically recognizes tumors, antigens and circulating products of such tumors (e.g., α-fetoprotein and hCG in testicular cancer and carcino-embryonic antigen in colorectal cancer). The detection of the antigen/antibody reaction can be effected with a color reaction (dye), a radioactive marker, an enzyme electrode, or by simply observing agglutination. The technique for producing monoclonal antibodies (MABs) in vivo and in vitro is well established since their discovery in 1974 by George Kohler and Cesar Milstein. More than 200 MAB systems are available commercially for research and some 50 MAB kits are now on the market or are close to FDA approval.

Diagnostic Test

Immunodiagnostics are now 20% of a $250 million U.S. medical diagnostic industry. The in vitro diagnosis market is estimated at $1 billion in 1990, when 50% of all the diagnostic tests will be based on monoclonal antibodies.

Some of the commercially available or soon to be available MAB systems include:

Prostatic Acid Phosphatase (PAP)	Abbott Lab., Hybritech
Pregnancy test (hCG hormone)	Monoclonal Antibodies, Inc.
T and B lymphocytes, monocytes, leukocyte	Johnson & Johnson
Viral Hepatitis	Centocor, Inc.
Pancreatic, gastric, colorectal cancers	Centrocor, Inc.
Carcinoembryonic antigen (CEA)	Abbott Lab.
Plant Viruses	American Type Culture Collection
Ferritin	Hybritech
Immunoglobulin E	Hybritech
Prolactin	Hybritech
Growth hormone	Hybritech
Rheumatic fever susceptibility	Rockefeller Univ.
Protein Myosin	Mass. Gen. Hosp.
Hodgkins disease	Albrecht Univ., FRG
Salmonella	Immunocell Corp.
Respiratory diseases diagnosis	Genetic Systems Corp.

(continued)

Pneumonia	
Cold	
Legionnaire's disease	
Gonorrhea, syphilis, cytomegalo-virus, varicella zoster, chlamydia, herpes	Genetic Systems Corp.
Different human blood cells	Genetic Systems Corp.
Anti-A anti-B	Celltech, Ltd.
Leukemia, breast, lung, colon, prostate cancers	Genetic Systems, Oncogen
Radioactive MAB (cancer treatment)	Nuclear & Genetic Technology
Human T cell leukemia virus	Biotech Research Lab.
Human proteins (Ig's, etc.)	Serotex

Biological Imaging

It is relatively straightforward to prepare "hot antibodies," that is antibodies labeled with a radioisotope. Such labeled antibodies can be used to identify, locate, and define a variety of sites, tissues, and cell populations [4]. The major application is the identification of tumor masses prior to treatment. Using gamma gamera it is possible to develop an image of the mass of interest.

Other applications are possible. For instance, at Massachusetts General Hospital, monoclonal antibody, to the protein myosin, labeled with radioactive technetium-99m allows to visualize damaged area in the heart muscle following heart attacks [5].

DNA PROBES

Three thousand three hundred sixty-eight discrete genetic disorders are known. In some 300 cases, the mechanism is understood. Although most such diseases are quite rare (an exception is hypercholesterolemia which hits one in 500 in the U.S.), they add up to about 10% of the total number of diseases affecting us [6]. In a number of cases the sequence of the gene involved is well-known and the mutated base pairs well identified, (e.g., β^{39}-globin in thalassaemia). It is then possible to design a DNA probe suitably labeled to hunt for such markers. This is already possible for such diseases as sickle cell anaemia (1 in every 520 blacks in the U.S. is affected), thalassaemia, Lesch-Nyhan syndrome, Huntington's chorea (20,000 Americans afflicted), and phenylketouria (incidence of 1 in 1,400 live births) [7–12]. A form of diarrhea-causing bacteria has been detected by a DNA probe in human samples. Possible in the very near future would be the detection of haemophilia (factor VII, VII, IX), coagulation factor IX, and Duchenne muscular dystrophy.

The requirements for using a DNA probe based on the blot-hybridization technique originally described by Southern [13] include:

- The nucleotide sequence of the gene must be known.
- A genetic DNA probe—some 20 nucleotides in length—matching the defect portion of the gene is synthetized.
- A label—normally phosphorus 32—is attached to some of the nucleotides.
- The DNA is digested with a restriction endonuclease (such enzymes cut the DNA at specific clevage sites).
- Electrophoresis of the mixture is performed on agarose gel.
- The DNA fragments are denatured making them single stranded and transferred to a nitrocellulose sheet. The sheet is then exposed to the labeled probe.
- The probe reacts with DNA strains from the patient. The probes will bind to the DNA strain only if it is its perfect complement.
- After washing away the rest of the radioactive DNA, autoradiography reveals the position and hence the size of the DNA fragment.

For example, single cell anemia is associated with a single mutation at position 6 (valine for glutamine) in β-globin. The endonuclease Mst II recognizes CCTGAGG coding for amino acids 5 to 7 in normal β-globin while sickle β-globin with sequence CCTGTGG is not recognized by the endonuclease. This allows to differentiate the sickle cell β-globin from normal human globin [14].

Traditionally the probe is labeled with radioactive species. Now comes a new technique making the probe so much sharper [15]. The idea is to replace the radioisotope with a "reporter" molecule: biotin. The presence of biotin is detected by avidin in a color reaction. Greatly enhanced sensitivity is achieved.

A number of viruses have been detected by DNA probes: hepatitis Virus [14], Epstein-Baar virus and cytomegalovirus [16]. The technique appears promising, with the necessary care, to detect a variety of genetic diseases and viral diseases. The technique should also be applicable to detecting a variety of oncogenes [17]. Eventually the technique could lead to early diagnosis and treatment of many more genetic diseases such as diabetes, muscular dystrophy, multiple sclerosis, and even cancer [18].

Union officials and workers worry about the implication of such a technique as a screening test for employees working under conditions possibly hazardous to health; potentially affecting their ability to earn substantial wages [19]. Federal legislation and regulations cannot be far behind.

VACCINES

It is estimated that the use of vaccines has expanded our life span by some 15 years. Seven vaccines are commonly used in the U.S.: polio, diphtheria, whooping cough, tetanus, mumps, measles, and rubella. A variety of other vaccines are under development and tests. Little had changed since the 18th century when the English surgeon, Edward Jenner, prepared the first vaccine against smallpox, until the advent of biotechnology.

The Logic of Vaccination

The polio epidemic in the United States reached 58,000 cases in 1957. In 1977 only 17 cases were reported, showing the efficacy of both the Sabin and Salk vaccines. A recent attempt to immunize 200,000 people in 209 villages in India against tuberculosis (via BCG vaccine) was a total failure.

When it comes to vaccinations, strong feelings come to the surface and the arguments for and against take an acid form. The debate takes many forms: the live versus dead virus vaccine; the injected versus the oral vaccine; the number of deaths due to the infecting agent versus the number of deaths associated with vaccination; the level of vaccination coverage needed. Different infections behave differently; and different vaccines behave differently as a function of age, level of sanitation, population group, etc. [20]. In the U.S. the goal is now to achieve levels of immunization above 90% for all childhood diseases that can be prevented by vaccination.

Vaccines are one of the most effective and safe methods to prevent diseases. Already smallpox and measles have essentially been eradicated through their systematic use.

Production

The worldwide market for vaccines is about $2 billion/year creating intensive competition among the traditional vaccines manufacturers and the newer biotechnology firms.

Synthetic vaccines are made from short sequences (as few as six bases) carefully selected from surface proteins to include the characteristic shape that the antibody is likely to recognize [21]. The promise of synthetic vaccine is to do away with the need to compose vaccines from inactivated or attenuated strains of pathogenic microorganisms; and to actively avoid the necessity of a source of biological material (such as human blood, or cells) [22]. The production of bacterial and viral vaccines is quite different; the latest requiring a cell substrate [23]. The fear of vaccination, based on whole pathogens is associated with the rare incidence of shock, inflammation to the brain, and the disease itself. Additionally, synthetic vaccines are likely to be more stable [24].

The process could be generally characterized as follows:

Step 1: Determine the composition (base pairs, amino acids) of the proteins on the pathogen surface;

Step 2: Identify base on principles, computer modeling techniques or mutant organisms, the subunit essential for recognition by the antibodies [25];

Step 3: Synthesize the subunit. The genetic material (once injected in a bacterium) can now serve as instruction for producing many copies of the active region.

It is the prevailing theory that proteins must be fairly large to initiate immune response. Subunit epitops can be attached to a carrier protein or to liposomes. Peptides with differing specificities might be coupled to a single carrier to give a multivalent vaccine [26].

The remaining problems include antigenic variability requiring new synthetic peptides for each strain. This should not be such a major problem with current sequencing methods and synthetic techniques [26].

A Sexist Vaccine

In spite of astral arrangements, diet, exercise, and a variety of positions; nature produces about the same number of boys and girls at birth (actually the ratio is 105 boys for 100 girls). Studies in the 1970s by anthropologists in tribes in the Senegal and Eskimo populations, brought to the attention of the world a dramatic change in the ratio: sometimes heavily in favor of girls, sometimes heavily in favor of boys. Painstaking detective work uncovered a correlation between viral hepatitis and sexes repartition at birth.

The phenomenon is explained as follows: The antigen Australia (the name given to the hepatitis type B virus antigen) is very similar in structure to the HY antigen (the antigen on the surface of spermatozoids Y).

It should be remembered that spermatozoids came in two forms: spermatozoids X (with an X chromosome) leading to the birth of females, and spermatozoids Y (with a Y chromosome) leading to the birth of males. This similarity between the Australian antigen and the HY antigen would foster cross immunologic reactions. People bearing the Australian antigen would produce more boys because of an increased tolerance of their immune system to the HY antigens.

Based on the findings, it should be possible to develop a vaccine specifically destroying the Y spermatozoids, favoring the birth of girls or the X spermatozoids with the consequent birth of boys.

A Vaccine Against Cancer

Malignant meloma is a fatal form of skin cancer. Scientists at Emory University in Atlanta have achieved 88% success by injecting a new vaccine under the skin of patients following surgery to remove the lymph nodes. The vaccine is made from cancer cells and a virus not normally causing disease in humans. It is postulated that a viral antigen is introduced on the cell surface, by the virus, close to a tumor antigen. The presence of the tumor antigen in some way enhances the action of the cellular antigen; stimulating the immune system to hunt for tumor cells.

A Birth Control Vaccine

A large effort goes into research and development to engineer better birth control methods: more effective, longer lasting, minimum side effect, applicable to both sexes, etc.

A number of efforts have departed from the traditional route and are aiming at developing a sterilizing vaccine. Researchers at the University of Saskatchewan are developing a system to neutralize the reproductive cycle. It works by neutralizing the effect of the hypothalamic gonadothoprin releasing hormone (GnRH). This releasing factor normally stimulates the pituitary to release a number of hormones responsible for triggering sexual maturation: release of eggs in females and spermatozoids in males. The vaccine is made up by linking a piece of GnRH with a compound known to stimulate the immune system. The immune system then recognizes both the inserted GnRH and that normally produced by the hypothalamus as foreign agents and neutralizes them. Tests in animals have achieved sterility up to two years with occasional booster injections.

Researchers at Northwestern University are working on a different birth control vaccine. The enzyme lactate dehydrogenase C_4 (LDH C_4) is naturally produced in the testes and is found on the surface of sperms. A synthetic peptide fragment, synthetized by the scientists, has antigenic activity comparable to the intact LDH C_4 enzyme. When injected in females it produces antibodies that prevent conception. The experimental vaccines appears to prevent fertility for several months. When the antibody level drops below a certain level, fertility returns.

Vaccines Against the Diseases of Man

Genetic engineering is being applied to developing a variety of vaccines against severe diseases.

Hepatitis

Over 250 million people carry the hepatitis B disease. It is a debilitating disease leading to chronic liver disease as well as cancer (hepato cellular carcinoma) and may cause premature death. An effective vaccine prepared from the infected blood of Americans (it consists of part of the virus coat—hepatitis B surface antigen) is available from Merck at around $100 a dose. The need to develop a cheaper vaccine has stimulated a race between American, French, British, Swiss and Dutch firms. One fascinating approach is to modify vaccinia, the cowpox virus, to make a vaccine against hepatitis B using genetic engineering. Scientists have been successful in inserting the gene for HbsAg into vaccinia. The modified vaccinia produced antigens in cell culture but also provided immunity to the virus when injected into rabbits. The problem with this solution is prior success in the smallpox vaccination program. Today, most of the Third World is immune to vaccinia, which would not flourish long enough to produce hepatitis antigen. This is not an insurmountable problem; with advances in genetic engineering, vaccinia could probably be sufficiently modified to get around this problem as well as the always present danger associated with vaccinia immunization. It is not farfetched to postulate a series of attenuated viruses colonizing the mucous membranes of the intestinal or respiratory tracts and releasing their antigens into the blood stream [27–29].

Malaria

It is estimated that 200 million or more people living in underdeveloped tropical areas suffer from malaria. In spite of early success of DDT on the *Anopheles* mosquitoes and drugs on the *Plasmodium* parasites, the incidence of malaria is on the rise.

Four species cause malaria in humans [30]. The four major stages: sporozoite, exoerythrocytic forms, blood forms and gametocytes all have quite different surface antigens [31]. The problem of developing a vaccine becomes a challenging one. It is now quite clear that intact parasites whether attenuated or killed will not serve as the active agent of a vaccine. Since the surface protein from sporozoites is similar in all species examined; this stage becomes the logical target. Progress so far has indicated that it is possible to identify potential antigen, to clone the DNA involved to produce the peptides, and to synthetize these peptides artificially [32].

Herpes

British scientists from the Birmingham University's Medical School have developed a herpes (based on killed viruses) vaccine. It seems to be quite effective with no observed side effects. It is not clear which strains of herpes would respond to the vaccine. A number of American firms are pursuing genetically engineered herpes vaccines: Molecular Genetics, Inc./Lederle and Merck and Company.

Flu

Influenza is one of the most common recurring diseases. Killed viruses are ineffective and live viruses only cause the disease. Scientists at the National Institutes of Health have engineered a vaccine made up of a gene controlling the virus' ability to multiply from a bird strain and the gene from the human virus controlling the development of the virus' antigens. The virus resulting from the mating of the bird (without the antigens) and human viruses (with the antigen) multiplies readily but does not cause the disease. It carries both the haemagglutinin and neuroamidase antigens important in stimulating the production of protective antibodies [33].

Gonorrhea

A vaccine based on hairlike structures on the gonococcus-bacterium surface was developed at the University of Pittsburgh.

Other

Vaccines based on viral subunits are already on the market. Vaccines for two types of meningitis and one type of pneumonia have faired well.

Animal Vaccines

Because of a shortened approval cycle and the lack of dominance by major pharmaceutical firms, many companies are developing vaccines for animal care (pets and farm animals). Originally most efforts are directed at viral vaccines but eventually similar activity will follow for bacterial, helmintic, etc., vaccines.

The most notable activities in this field are foot and mouth disease and pig scour vaccines (affecting 15% of newborn pigs), rabies, and distemper in pets and a vaccine to prevent coccidiosis in poultry (costing some $300 million a year in losses to broiler suppliers in the U.S.) [34,35].

In the case of animal vaccines, the dose schedule and the duration of immunization is all important. Because of the logistic and practical difficulties in vaccinating animals, a single dose protection is ideal.

ANTIBIOTICS

History

Antibiotics are synonymous with success in the pharmaceutical industry. In 1941 penicillin entered human therapeutics. By 1944 the use of penicillin was widely adopted by allied armies in World War II. Cephalosporins were derived from a fungus found in 1945 in a sewage outlet in Sardinia. These antibiotics entered the market in 1958-1959. Azactam was recently derived from a molecule discovered in swampy soil in New Jersey. New antibiotics are discovered every year.

Market

The worldwide market for antibiotics is around $1.6 billion. One company owns 40% of that market. The Cephalosporin family (the antibiotic market can be split in broad categories: penicillin and its derivatives; aminoglycosides; and cephalosporins) represent a $700 million slice of that market.

The cost of bringing a new product to the market is forever increasing; it is now estimated at $50 million to $75 million. It is a risky business from disappointing technical results, to lawsuits, to the looming Japanese competition; but it is a financially rewarding business.

Resistance

Antibiotics of the β-lactam group act on bacteria by disrupting the cell wall synthesis mechanism through the inhibition of enzymes involved in cross-linking D-alanyl peptides on peptidoglycan strands of growing cells [36].

In 1946, 14% of isolated staphylococcus were resistant to penicillin; in 1947, 38%; in 1948, 59%; in 1950 the majority of "staph" hospital infections were associated with resistant strains, in 1982, 80 to 90% of isolated staphylococcus were resistant. Today we observe an epidemic of bacterial resistance to antibiotics. How does this resistance arise?

Bacteria produce a variety of enzymes: phosphorylases, adenylases, acetylases capable of attacking antibiotics. But no enzyme is more effective in their struggle for life than the β-lactamase which hydrolyses the amide linkage of the β-lactam rendering the drug impotent.

Another defense mechanism is the ability of bacteria to change the permeability of the membrane with a group of enzymes called permeases, blocking the entry of the antibiotics. Under selective pressure, bacteria have adapted to a variety of conditions. Unfortunately, bacteria have the uncanny ability to disseminate this acquired resistance to antibiotics by transfer of genes. Four mechanisms are at work:

- *Transduction*—The gene is incorporated into the virus (bacteriophage) infecting bacteria. The gene is integrated into the chromosome.
- *Transformation*—Direct transfer of gene (cell free DNA) from one bacteria to another.
- *Conjugation*—Direct transfer between donor and recipient cells.
- *Fusion*—The fusion of two cells.

To each weapon there is a defense and to each defense there is a better weapon. Scientists have not thrown in the towel.

New Vogue of Antibiotics

A number of lines of attack are being pursued and strategies emerge [37].

- The preparation of an always expanding arsenal of antibiotics with a spectrum as large as possible for killing as many species of bacteria as possible.
- The preparation of more effective derivatives starting from the basic structure of penicillins and cephalosporins.
- The preparation of antibiotics resistant to -lactamases. Cefotaxime is a first born in the cephalosporin family with this property. The monobactam group is providing many new candidates.
- The elimination from the antibiotic molecule of the fragment susceptible to the bacterial enzyme. Some success has been achieved in the aminoside family (of which streptomycine is a member). This ap-

proach, unfortunately, fails for the penicillin since the antibiotic active site and the vulnerable site are the same.

- Clavulanic acid produced by *Streptomyces claviligerus* has the unique ability to inactivate irreversibly the penicillase enzymes. A pharmaceutical preparation containing two-thirds penicillin and one-third clavulanic acid, called "augmentin" has been tested with success.

The Role of Biotechnology

The production of antibiotics is partially an art, and partially a science. Our state of knowledge on the production of antibiotics has matured, although much of this knowledge is privately held [38–41]. Hydrophobic penicillins can be produced by a variety of species of fungus. *Penicillium chrysogenum* is the species usually chosen for industrial production [40,42]. Hydrophilic β-lactam antibiotics such as penicillin and cephalosphorins are produced by fungi such as *Cephalosporium* and actinomycetes. A new group of antibiotics—monobactams have been produced by *Pseudomonas, Acetobacter, Chromobacterium* and *Agrobacterium*.

The microbial synthesis of antibiotics is regulated by the source of carbon, nitrogen, phosphorus and specific amino acids, typically, lysine and methionine [39]. Production of antibiotics is optimized under conditions of nutrient imbalance and low growth rates. Important efforts are underway to optimize both the fermentation process and the product recovery phase. Only 10% of the glucose goes toward penicillin production, and half the manufacturing cost is associated with product recovery [41].

INTERFERON

What Is Interferon?

Interferon is very much like nuclear fusion. It has been called the ultimate weapon. It is a molecule that fascinates and passionates the layman and the scientist. It dissatifies by its results only to give rise to a new vague of interest, often in a new direction.

Some 25 years ago Isaacs and Lindenmann discovered that animal cells infected with a virus collected a protein interfering with further viral infection. They called this secreted protein—*interferon*.

A bewildering variety of effects have been ascribed to interferon at the cellular level [43]. Inhibition of cell division and tumor growth, enhancement of phagocytosis of macrophages, cytotoxicity of lymphocytes, activity of natural killer cells and production of antibodies.

Interferon is present in all vertebrates and is species specific. Human interferon have been grouped into three major classes: IFN-α (leukocyte), IFN-β (fibroblast) and IFN-γ (immune).

More information is accumulating every day on the molecular structure of interferon. All interferons are proteins made up of 146 to 166 amino acids. The first 20 or so (at the NH2 terminal) are a signal peptide which is hydrolyzed during production. During their synthesis the β and γ interferons have multiple lateral chains. These are not necessary for the antiviral action of interferon. Based on experimental work we can conclude that the 17 first amino acids are essential to the activity of human interferon. Cysteine bonds, playing a central role in the spatial folding of proteins are essential to the activity of the protein.

How Does It Work

The ability of interferon to prevent viral infection is the best understood of all the actions of interferon. Many substances can induce cells to produce interferon: bacteria, antibiotics, lipopolysaccharides and especially double-stranded RNA's. The mechanism of interferon induction probably resembles the classical induction system well studied in bacteria where an inducer turns on the interferon gene by removing a repressor that was preventing its expression [44].

Once the interferon molecules are synthetized, they diffuse out of the cells. When interferon binds to the surface of a susceptible cell, it triggers a complex chain of events.

We now know that the antiviral action of interferon is mediated by the synthesis of specific proteins. One protein is a protein kinase, that is an enzyme involved in the transfer of a phosphate group from ATP to an acceptor protein. The second protein catalyzes the formation of a very unusual compound ppp A2′p52′p5′A (p=phosphate). This compound is a nuclease activator that activates the third protein, an endonuclease that breaks down RNA's.

The production of interferon by lymphocytes is especially interesting. The lymphocytes like many other cells, release interferon when stimulated by viral inducers. They also produce immune interferon when exposed to mitogens or to specific antigens. Under these conditions they release a family of mediating substances called lymphokines [45].

The anti-cancer effect of interferon is most likely due to the molecule activating the normal body defenses, for instance by stimulating the natural killer (NK) cells to destroy malignant cells.

The State of Affairs

A clear picture of the therapeutic effect of interferon has been long to develop. It has been difficult to produce enough of the pure compound for large scale testing. Some 10–14 α interferons are produced in the body, to say nothing of β and γ interferons; complicating the picture [46]. Interferons have many properties, including an hormone-like behavior. Interferons act directly but also boost other normal functions such as NK cells activity or the production of antibodies. The complexity of interferon in structure, function, and action is becoming apparent.

Based on clinical trials, interferon appears to be the body's first line of defense against infection by many viruses [45]. Interferon is unlikely to be useful in a preventive mode since the effects of interferon are transient and the attended protection vanishes within very few days [43].

Encouraging results have been obtained with alpha and beta interferons in the local treatment of herpes labilis, herpes zosters and cytomegalovirus. A measure of success has been achieved in the treatment of certain cancers: multiple myeloma, breast cancer, lymphoma and osteosarcoma [47]. $2'5A$ is a potent inhibitor of protein synthesis. A modified version is being tested against herpes [48]. The use of interferon is not without side effects. Reports of abnormal brain waves, lethargy and severe confusion have surfaced.

Biotechnology and Interferon Production

At least 30 firms and organizations are in the interferon business. Large pharmaceutical firms and chemical corporations such as Bristol-Myers Company, Burroughs-Wellcome Co., Du Pont de Nemour and Company, Hoffman-La Roche, Schering-Plough Corporation, Abbott Laboratories, and Searle and Co.; specialized companies such as Interferon, Inc., Lee Biomolecular Research Labs, Inc., National Geno Sciences, Inc.; and biotechnology companies like Cetus, Biogen, Genentech, Inc., are all involved [49,50].

Biogen was the first firm to clone the human interferon in the bacteria *E. coli* and get it to function [51]. *E. coli* is not a very good vector for secreting protein. Only 20% of the interferon produced by the cell is secreted. Of this 20%, 10% is free in the medium. *Bacillus subtilis* is a better secretor and the organism transformed with a plasmid bearing the interferon gene, will secrete the protein. Recently, attention has turned to the yeast *Saccharomyces cerevisiae*; since we know so much more about fermentation it might be the organism of choice [52]. A great deal of work is going on in improving yield, developing new strains and working with pro-interferon. The race is on [53,54].

HORMONES

Some 40 hormones are of importance to man's health. These are listed in Table 7-1, indicating origin, target tissue and major physiological actions [55,56].

Biotechnologies have been applied to producing a number of hormones, only two will be reviewed.

Insulin

Eli Lilly controls 80% of the domestic market for insulin. The source of insulin for the 1.5 million diabetics in the U.S. is swine and cattle pancreatic glands. Genentech/Eli Lilly is the first company to produce bacterially cloned insulin—humulin. The synthetic insulin is targeted to the $137 million/year domestic insulin market [57].

Novo Industry and E.R. Squibb use a different approach to make insulin for human use. Starting with readily available swine insulin, they enzymatically change the one amino acid that distinguishes it from human insulin [58].

Growth Hormone

In 1976, Biogen succeeded in cloning human growth hormone in bacteria. Prior to this achievement, the hormone was extracted from the pea-size pituitary of cadavers. Because of the size of the hormone, 19,000 daltons; this is a most significant achievement.

Growth hormone is important in the treatment of pituitary deficient children. The hormone might also be valuable in healing burns, wounds, bleeding ulcers, broken bones and in combatting osteoporosis.

In Sweden, a bacterially produced form of hGH is named somatoniam. It differs from human growth hormone by having an extra methionine group at the end of the 191 amino acid long molecule.

Other Hormones

Recombinant DNA techniques are systematically being applied to the mass production of a number of hormones.

TABLE 7-1. Important Hormones.

Endocrine Organ	Hormone	Source	Target Tissue	Major Physiological Actions
Anterior pituitary	Growth hormone	Acidophilic cells	All tissues	Stimulates general body growth
	Adrenocorticotropin (ACTH)	Unknown	Adrenal cortex	Maintenance of function of adrenal cortex
	Thyrotropin (TSH)	Small basophilic cells	Thyroid	Stimulate secretion of thyroxine
	Prolactin (LTH)	Acidophilic cells	Ovaries and mammary gland	Corpus luteum maintenance and progesterone secretion in some species, milk secretion
	Luteinizing hormone (LH)	Large basophilic cells	Ovaries and testes	Androgen secretion by testes, maturation of follicles and ovulation
	Follicle stimulating hormone (FSH)	Large basophilic cells	Ovaries and testes	Oogenesis and spermatogenesis
Intermediate lobe of pituitary	Melanocyte stimulating hormone (MSH)	Basophilic cells	Melanophore cells	Controls cutaneous pigmentation
Posterior pituitary	Oxytocin	Supraoptic and paraventricular nuclei of hypothalamus	Mammary gland and uterus	Milk release and contraction of uterus
	Vasopressin	Supraoptic and paraventricular nuclei of hypothalamus	Peripheral blood vessels and kidney tubules	Constriction of blood vessels and water absorption from kidney tubules

(continued)

TABLE 7-1. (continued).

Endocrine Organ	Hormone	Source	Target Tissue	Major Physiological Actions
Thyroid	Thyroxine and triiodothyronine	Thyroid follicles	All tissue	Increased rate of cellular metabolism
	Calcitonin	Ultimobranchial cells	Bone, kidney	Decreases blood calcium levels
Parathyroid	Parathyroid hormone	Chief cells	Bone, kidney and intestine	Increases blood calcium levels
Adrenal cortex	Glucocorticoids	Zona fasiculata and zona reticularis	All tissues	Mobilizes body energy sources, increase blood sugar levels, antiflammatory action
	Mineralocorticoids	Zona glomerulosa	Kidney, all tissues indirectly	Salt and water balance
Adrenal medulla	Epinephrine	Chromaffin cells	Heart, skeletal muscle and liver	Increases strength of heart contraction and heart rate, increases blood sugar
	Norepinephrine	Chromaffin cells	Peripheral blood vessels, smooth muscle	Constriction of peripheral vessels and contraction of smooth muscles and glands
Pancreas	Glucagon	Alpha cells of Islet of Langerhans	Liver	Raises blood sugar levels
	Insulin	Beta cells of Islet of Langerhans	Muscle and adipose tissue	Lowers blood sugar levels
Kidney	Renin and angiotensin	Juxtaglomerular cells	Zona glomerulosa	Increases blood pressure, aldosterone secretion
Ovary	Estrogens	Follicles	Mammary gland,	Stimulates development and maintenance of

(continued)

TABLE 7-1. (continued).

Endocrine Organ	Hormone	Source	Target Tissue	Major Physiological Actions
	Progesterone	Corpus leteum	Mammary gland, genital tract	female secondary sexual characteristics Required for implantation of fetus
	Relaxin	Unknown	Cartilage and ligaments of pelvic girdle	Relaxation of cartilage and ligaments to facilitate parturition
Testes	Androgens	Interstitial cells	Accessory sex organs, testes	Development of accessory sex organ and secondary sex characteristics of male
Gastrointestinal tract	Secretin	Pyloric mucosa of stomach	Pancreas	Stimulates alkaline secretion for digestion
	Pancreozymin	Mucosa of duodenum	Pancreas	Stimulates enzyme secretion for digestion
	Cholecystokinin (CCK)	Mucosa of duodenum	Gall bladder	Evacuates bile into intestine
	Enterogastrone	Mucosa of duodenum	Stomach	Inhibits motility and acid secretion of stomach
	Gastrin	Mucosa of duodenum	Stomach	Stimulates secretion of HCl
Hypothalamus	Tyrotropin releasing factor (TRP)		Pituitary	Secretion of thyrotropin and prolactin
	Corticotropin re-leasing factor (CRF)		Pituitary	Control secretion of corticotropin

(continued)

TABLE 7-1. (continued).

Endocrine Organ	Hormone	Source	Target Tissue	Major Physiological Actions
	Growth hormone releasing factor (GHRF)		Pituitary	Control secretion of growth hormone
	Prolactin release inhibiting factor (PRIF)		Pituitary	Control secretion of prolactine
	Luteinising hormone releasing factor (LHRH)		Pituitary	Control release of LH
Placenta	Placental lactogene (PL)			Lactogen action
	Chorionic gonado-tropin (hCG)	Syncytiotrophoblast	Corpus luteum	Secretion of estrogen and progestine
Urogenital tract	Urogastrone Myotonin			

Source: Modified from Ref. 55.

- Genentech, Inc. has a patent for producing the brain hormone, somatostatin.
- Serono Laboratories is attempting to transfer genes from placenta and pituitary gland cells into *E. coli*, yeasts and mammalian cells, hoping to induce these cells to express folicle stimulating hormones (FSH), luteinizing hormone (LH) and chorionic gonadotropin (hCG).
- A company is offering for sale the synthetic gene coding for human pancreatic growth hormone-releasing factor (hpGRF).
- Tumors secrete hormones. This has led to the establishment of a number of hormone secreting animal and human cell lines for ACTH, growth hormone, prolactin, and gonadotrophin [59].

GROWTH FACTORS

A growing number of growth factors are appearing on the scene (Table 7-2) [60].

TABLE 7-2. Some Protein and Peptide "Growth Factors" with Potential Pharmaceutical Applications.

Factor		Function
CSF	Colony stimulating factors	Stimulate granulocyte differentiation
ECGS	Endothelial cell growth supplement	Required by cells from vascular lining
EDGF	Endothelial-derived growth factor	Stimulates cell division in blood vessels
EGF	Epidermal growth factor	Stimulates growth of epidermal cells and many tumors
FGF	Fibroblast growth factor	Stimulates fibroblast cell growth
FN	Fibronectin	Stimulates adhesion and proliferation
MDGF	Macrophage-derived growth factor	Stimulates division near inflammation
NGF	Nerve growth factor	Stimulates nerve growth and repair
PDGF	Platelet-derived growth factor	Stimulates division of fibroblast-like cells
SGF	Skeletal growth factor	Stimulates bone cell growth
WAF	Wound angiogenesis factor	Stimulates wound healing
TAF	Tumor angiogenesis factor	Blood vessel proliferation in tumors
IGFI IGFII	Insulin-like growth factor (somatomedins I and II)	Intermediates in control of tissue growth
TGGF	T-cell growth factor	Long-term growth of T cells
BCGF	B-cell growth factor	Short-term proliferation of B-cells
SF	Spreading factor	Promote spreading of cells in cultures

Source: Modified from Ref. 60–65.

Retroviruses have arisen by the substitution of viral material necessary for replication with segment of host genetic information. When incorporated into the retroviral genome, these onc genes have the ability to induce neoplastic transformation [61]. Cells transformed by retroviruses and cells stimulated by growth factors have striking similarities. When the Simian sarcoma virus (SSV) onc gene v-vis was compared to platelet derived growth factor (PDGF) important structural homology and immunological similarities were observed [61,62]. PDGF are potent mitogenic proteins. They are also chemoattractant for human neutrophiles and monocytes. They are well suited to mediate inflammatory and repair processes and may play a role in the genesis of artherosclerosis [62].

Transforming growth factors (TGF) secreted by humans have many of the same biological properties as epidermal growth form (EGF); among others they stimulate bone resorption [63]. Transforming growth factors is a heterogeneous group of low molecular weight polypeptides characterized by their ability to induce transformed phenotype [64]. They have been found in almost all tissue neoplastic and non neoplastic and in many different species.

The potential medical applications are many: correction of dwarfism, speeding the growth of premature infants, the treatment of burn victims. These growth factors are currently not produced by biotechnology, but extracted from cells and tissues [65–69].

PLASMA PROTEINS

More than 100 proteins have been isolated from human blood plasma [70]. These proteins are of interest because of their prophylactic and therapeutic properties, as reagents for clinical diagnosis, and as model to elucidate the function of proteins at the molecular level. Their concentration in human plasma vary widely from 4g/100 ml for albumin to 5 mg/100 ml for IgE, the average being around 100 mg/100 ml.

A number of key proteins with prophylactic and therapeutic actions and the clinical indication for their use are given below.

Protein	Indication
Gamma globulin	Antibody deficiency
Albumin	Volume substitute
Fibrinogen (Factor I)	Abnormal bleeding
Immunoglobins	Antibody deficiencies

(continued)

Protein	Indication
Prothrombin (Factor II)	Hemophilia B
Factor IX	Hemophilia B
Transferrin	Inborn deficiencies
Plasminogen	Fibrinolysis therapy
Factor F XIII	Abnormal bleeding
C1 Inactivator	Angioneurotic edema
α-antitrypsin	Pulmonary emphysema
Christmas factor (Factor IX)	Abnormal bleeding
Proconvertin (Factor VII)	Abnormal bleeding
Antihemophilic globulin (Factor VIII)	Hemophilia A
β-lipoprotein	Neuromuscular distrophy

A great deal of interest in the clotting system (some 14 protein components, not counting inhibitors) the complement system, proteinase inhibitors, immunoglobins, lipoproteins, and carrier proteins is translated in attempts at producing them by recombinant DNA techniques as an alternative to the traditional plasma fractionation.

THE CONTROL OF REPRODUCTION

The methods for the control of reproduction have evolved from physical devices, to chemical molecules, to biotechnology derived concepts. They have evolved from a concentration on the female reproductive system to an attack on both sexes. They have evolved from a single prone approach to an arsenal of weapons from hormones to vaccines.

Billions of women are seeking a better alternative to the pill and a number of men would be interested in an alternative to vasectomy. A new class of contraceptive based on the use of analogues of luteinizing hormone releasing hormone (LHRH) is innocent of side effects and is rapidly inactivated. These analogues inhibit reproductive functions by decreasing the LHRH stimulus to the anterior pituitary responsible for modulating the release of luteinizing hormone (LH) and follicle-stimulating hormone (FSH). LHRH injected in man decreases sperm production. Unfortunately, testosterone levels in blood also declines. It is hoped that with appropriate modification, one function (sperm reduction) can be enhanced where the other (testosterone reduction) is avoided [71,72].

The same LHRH hormone also has a role in treating precocious puberty, suppressing sexual development until the appropriate age. One in every 5,000 to 10,000 children is affected with this distressing abnormality. Human menopausal gondrotropin (hMG) has proven useful in treating female and male infertility. Many efforts are underway to probe the control of the ovarian and testicular function. More polypeptides will be identified and their role documented. Eventually they will reach the arsenal of birth control chemicals inexorably moving toward using the tools that nature has built.

The implication of these findings is that biotechnology will play an increasing role in developing methods for large scale production of such hormones controlling the reproduction cycle.

THERAPY

The possibility of using enzymes in therapy is well established and practiced for a small set of enzymes. The use of bifunctional antibody in therapy is rapidly gaining favor. The fascinating and ultimate therapy is gene therapy.

Enzyme Therapy

Enzymes have been used in a solubilized form or immobilized on some substrates; they have been given orally, injected or implanted in soft tissue as prostheses; and they also have been used in extracorporeal equipment [73].

To be used *in vivo*, enzymes must meet stringent requirements:

- The enzyme must be larger than 60,000 daltons to avoid immediate glomerular filtration and excretion in urine;
- They must be protected through encapsulation or immobilization to avoid denaturation and proteolysis;
- They must not activate immunological reactions;
- They must have high purity to insure efficacity and avoid side effects;
- They must be targeted; and
- Control over duration of physiological activity is required.

A few examples should give an idea of the range of possibilities of enzymes in therapy.

Hyaluronidase

This enzyme hydrolyses hyaluronic acid, a polysaccharide. The enzyme is used as a dispersion agent with injected drugs [74].

L-asparaginase

The enzyme is promising in the treatment of lymphoid leukosis. Certain kinds of leukemia require an exogenous source of asparagine for growth. The enzyme, L-asparaginase acts by hydrolyzing L-asparagine in the plasma, achieving tumor mass reduction [74].

In other tumors, glutamine is an important energy source. These same tumors are sensitive to the anticancer activity of glutamine antimetabolites (e.g., acivicin). The extreme toxicity of these compounds limit their use. By reducing the amount of glutamine available, lower doses of the antimetabolites can be used, achieving higher levels of tumor inhibition with lower density side effects. Tests are underway in animal systems [75].

Urease

Encapsulated urease has been tested in animals, upon oral ingestion for the removal of urea. Immobilized urease with ammonia absorbent is being used clinically in the dialysate regenerating system [76].

Alpha-1 Antitrypsin

The role of the protein alpha-1 antitrypsin (AAT) is to block the action of the digestive enzyme elastase. This enzyme destroys foreign matter entering the lung. Many emphysema victims suffer from a lack of AAT leading to elastase slowly destroying the lung tissue. Scientists have successfully isolated the human AAT gene and incorporated it in *E. coli* and in yeast for mass production. It still remains to test the idea that the AAT supplied externally would prevent further lung damage in emphysema victims.

Heparinase

Extracorporeal devices perfused with blood are commonly used in surgery and therapy. Their use requires heparinisation of the patient with the ever present possibility of hemorrhagic complications. A system using heparinase immobilized on a filter degrades heparin eliminating much of the difficulties [77].

Digestive Aid Enzymes

These enzymes (a mixture of enzymes) are largely used in Japan to aid digestion.

Fibrinolytic Agents

The obstruction of a blood vessel by a blood clot can have catastrophic effect. Thrombus have formed in the arterial and venous systems under a variety of conditions. The protein fibrin serves as a matrix to support the clot. The intent of fibrinolysis is to proteolytically degrade fibrin to a soluble product [78]. The human fibrinolytic system is complex and fine tuned. Streptokinase and urokinase are two enzymes involved in the activation of the endogeneous plasminogen system controlling the proteolytic action of plasmin on fibrin. Both enzymes have been used in the treatment of patients with blood clots. Tissue-type plasminogen activator has also been used to selectively remove clots [79–81].

Much effort is under way to produce such enzymes in large volume by cell culture [82] or by genetic engineering.

Anti-inflammatory Agents

Proteolytic enzymes have been used for the reduction of inflammation and edema. Their beneficial action is associated with the solution of fibrin and the clearing of proteinaceous debris. Bromelain, pancreatin, collagenase among others, have been used in this mode.

Collagen

Collagen is the major component of connective tissue. The physical and chemical nature of collagen can be readily modified. It is possible to cast collagen into a variety of shapes or into diverse surfaces. Collagen would be an ideal candidate for prostheses such as cornea, heart valves, blood vessels, etc. It has undergone tests as dialysis membranes and has proven beneficial in healing dermal wounds [82].

Enzyme Inducers

Maturity onset diabetes is associated with less than active enzymes in the liver. The limiting factor appears to be the speed at which glucose-6 phosphatase and glycogen synthetase do their work. Using enzyme inducers (phenobarbital and medroxyprogesterone acetate), it is possible to significantly reduce blood glucose, allowing a better control [84].

Enzyme Inactivator

A most fascinating potential therapeutic idea is the development of synthetic translation-inhibiting oligonucleotides-like polymers (STOP).

STOP molecule hybridizes with a disease-causing organism mRNA preventing the organism from making a specific protein. The idea has not yet been tested in realistic models [85].

The premise that inactivation of enzymes can be induced by misre-cognition of a substrate leads to the concept of suicidal substrates [86]. A number of cases have been documented, opening the door to new therapeutic actions.

Gene Therapy

Gene therapy could be applied to somatic line cells or to the germ line. The first has created considerable interest; the second, a great deal of controversey. Gene therapy can take several forms:

- Modification of existing genetic material (e.g., methylation-demethylation);
- Removal of genetic material (e.g., trisomies, sex chromosome anomalies);
- Addition of a genetic material.

Gene therapy is not feasible in humans now, although considerable success has been achieved in cells, tissue cultures, and animal models. Three major problems need to be resolved before wide scale application is possible: delivery of the gene to the target cell; the appropriate regulation of expression; and the safety of the gene to cell host. Five techniques have been practiced for gene delivery: viral, chemical (e.g., calcium phosphate precipitation), physical (e.g., microinjection), fusion (e.g., liposome, RBC ghost), and retroviral vectors. Expression can be improved by complex expression vectors. The safety of the gene has been established in a number of animal experiments.

Gene therapy is possibly the ultimate technique for correcting genetic errors. Experiments with animal models are promising. Scientists in France have been able to insert the preproinsuline gene in a bacterial plasmid and encapsulate it in liposome. Upon injection in rats, blood glucose levels drop significantly [87]. The -chains of homoglobin, when inserted into a mouse, produced human hemoglobin [88]. The gene for the enzyme thymidine kinase functioned when inserted in cells of a deficient mouse [88].

The introduction of genes into fertilized eggs has been attempted with success. Growth hormone genes, when introduced in rat and mouse cells, produce animals growing faster than without the gene.

For ethical reasons, it will be some time before the technique is perfected and dried on humans [89]. Attempts to try the technique in humans started a chorus of objections which has not died down yet [90].

Monoclonal Antibody Therapy

The great advantage of antibody in therapy is that they allow fine targeting, that is the delivery of the therapeutic agent to the intended sites.

Bifunctional antibodies have been used to target and deliver drugs, toxins, radioisotopes, liposomes and immunomodulating agents [91–98]. All cells contain surface markets. The same is true for cancer cells. This "address" can be used to target a monoclonal antibody carrying a toxic agent to kill such cells.

The basic problem in tumor therapy is to destroy malignant cells while minimizing damage to normal cells. In 1906 Paul Ehrlich, proposed the idea of a "magic bullet" that would have affinity for certain tissue and be a carrier of cytotoxic agents. Monoclonal antibodies reacting with tumor specific and associated antigens, are the modern counterpart of this dream.

One of the major problems with organ transplants is immuno rejection. Doctors at Mass. General Hospital use monoclonal antibodies directed against the T lymphocyte cells of the immune system involved in the process of rejection. Treatment of patients with kidney transplants brought about reversal of acute graph rejection in all cases [99].

Going further, scientists have developed a monoclonal antibody to the I-A gene products of the immune response gene complex. They observed the suppression of the clinical manifestation of experimental autoimmune Myastheia gravis. This finding opens the door to the treatment of autoimmune diseases [100].

In a far reaching series of experiments in animals, scientists tricked the immune system in making autobodies against its own hormone, hence controlling growth, reproduction and metabolism [101]. Using modified hormones, they essentially immunized the animals against their own hormones.

These few examples point out the power and diversity of antibodies as target and delivery systems in therapy. Much progress, including applications to humans, is expected in the near future.

Other Applications

Enzymes can be used as detoxifying agents against barbituate overdose or cyanide poisoning, as substitution to correct genetic metabolic error (such as phenylketouria) and in the synthesis of lacking metabolites [102].

More complex immobilized and encapsulated multienzyme systems are the answer to many therapeutic needs. Additional oncolytic enzymes (similar to *L. asparginase*) are under development or tests (Neuraminidase, ribonuclease, carboxypeptidase, L. methioninase, L. tyrosinase, etc.) [103–105].

LAST WORD   If nobody said anything unless he knew what he was talking about, a ghastly hush would descend upon the earth.
—SIR ALAN HERBERT

The giant steps taken by biology in recent years can be ascribed to the availability of techniques, methods, equipment and instruments. The structure of DNA would not have been known without x-ray crystallography. DNA and RNA sequences would not be known without chromatography and electrophoresis.

New techniques for producing protein of use in diagnosis and therapy will alter the structure of the pharmaceutical industry. Already immuno diagnostic tests have changed the diagnostic segment of the industry replacing old techniques, developing new ones and generally giving impetus to what was an established field.

The last chapter on the role of biotechnology in pharmacy has not been written. At the pace we see new advances, it might never be writen.

Looking the future straight in the face: we are indeed on a technology threshold, in a transition period; moving from a period of engineering technology base to one of emulation of nature. We have come a full circle. Facing up to the future, we must remember that we owe to future generations to leave this valley not worse off than we found it.

This is the last word.

REFERENCES

1. Chisholm, R., "On the Trail of the Magic Bullet," *High Technology,* 57–63 (Jan. 1983).
2. "Monoclonals by the Million," *New Scientist,* 271 (28 July 1983).
3. Netzer, W., "New England Monoclonal Resources Set Up to Apply in vitro Hybridoma Method," *GEN,* 9 (March/April 1983).
4. Hnatowich, D. J., W. W. Layne, R. L. Childs, D. Lanteigne, M. A. Davis, T. W. Griffin, P. W. Doherty, "Radioactive Labelling of Antibody: A Simple and Efficient Method," *Science, 220,* 613–615 (1983).
5. "A Quick Test for Heart Damage," *Chemical Week,* 16 (Feb. 23).
6. Williamson, B., "Gene Therapy," *Nature, 298,* 416–418 (1982).
7. Pirasto, M., Y. Waikan, A. Cad, B. J. Conner, R. L. Teplitz, and R. B. Wallace, "Prenatal Diagnosis of -Thalassemia," *New England J. Med., 309* (5), 284–287 (1983).

8. Boehn, C., S. E. Antonarakis, J. A. Phillips, III, G. Stetten, and H. H. Kazazian, Jr., "Prenatal Diagnosis Using DNA Polymorphismis," *New England J. Med., 308* (18), 1054-1058 (1983).

9. Antonarakis, S., C. D. Boehm, P. S. W. Giardina, and H. H. Kazazian, Jr., "Non-Random Association of Polymorphic Restriction Sites in the -Globin Gene Cluster," *Proc. Natl. Acad. Sci., 79,* 137-141 (1982).

10. Rosenfeld, A., "The Heartbreak Gene," *Science 81,* 46-50 (Dec. 1981).

11. "Gene Probes May Spot Genes Missing from Embryos," *New Scientist,* 777 (16 June 1983).

12. "NICHD-Funded Scientist Develops Gene Test to Diganose PKU in Unborn Children," *The NIH Record* (1983).

13. Southern, E. M., "Detection of Specific Sequences Among DNA Fragments Separated by Gel Electrophoresis," *J. Mol. Biol., 98,* 503-517 (1975).

14. Kronenberg, H. M., "Looking at Genes," *New England J. Med., 307* (1), 50-51 (1982).

15. Lewin, R., "Genetic Probes Become Ever Sharper," *Science, 16,* 167 (Sept. 1983).

16. Chou, S. and T. C. Merigan, "Rapid Detection and Quantitation of Human Cytomegalovirus in Urine Through DNA Hybridization," *New England J. Medicine, 308* (16), 921-925 (1983).

17. Kronfiris, T. G., "The Emerging Genetics of Human Cancer," *New England J. Med., 309* (7), 404-409 (1983).

18. "A Way to Detect Birth Defects," *Chemical Week,* 19 (Jan. 26, 1983).

19. U.S. Congress, "Genetic Screening of Workers," Hearing before Subcommittee on Investigations and Oversight, 97th Congress, 2nd Session, No. 119 (June 22, 1982).

20. Anderson, R. and R. May, "The Logic of Vaccination," *New Scientist, 18,* 410-415 (November 1982).

21. Emini, E. A., B. A. Jameson, and E. Wimmer, "Pairing for and Induction of Anti-poliovirus Neutralizing Antibodies by Synthetic Peptides," *Nature, 304,* 699-703 (1983).

22. Newmark, P., "Will Peptides Make Vaccines," *Nature, 305,* 9 (1983).

23. Beale, A. J. and R. J. P. Harris, "Microbial Technology: Production of Vaccines," in *Microbial Technology: Current State, Future Prospects,* Cambridge Univ. Press, NY (1979).

24. Arnon, R. and M. Sela, "Les Antigenes et Vaccins Synthetiques," *La Recherche, 142,* 346-357 (1983).

25. Lerner, R. A., "Synthetic Vaccines," *Sci. Am., 249,* 66-75 (1983).

26. Beale, J., "Synthetic Peptides as the Basis for Future Vaccines," *Nature, 298,* 14-15 (1982).

27. Beale, A. J., "Hybrid Vaccinia Virus for Mass Hepatitis Immunization?" *Nature, 302,* 471-477 (1983).

28. "New Hepatitis Vaccine Developed," *New Scientist, 11,* 419 (August 1983).

29. "Making a Hepatitis Vaccine from Cowpox Virus," *New Scientist, 12,* 375 (May 1983).

30. "Vaccine Gene," *Sci. Amer., 248* (5), 93-95 (1983).

31. Cox, F. E. G., "The Long Road to a Malaria Vaccine," *New Scientist, 20,* 176 (October 1983).

32. Cox, F. E. G., "Cloning Genes for Antigens of *Plasmodium falciparum,*" *Nature, 304,* 13-14 (1983).

33. "Marriage of Viruses Produce a New Flu Vaccine," *New Scientist, 27,* 230 (January 1983).

34. "Genetically Engineered Vaccine for Pigs," *New Scientist, 20,* 779 (March 1982).

35. Brown, M. J., "Genentech's Food and Mouth Vaccine Could Find Major Markets after Third World Trials," *GEN,* 3 (Jan/Feb 1983).

36. Kelly, J. A., P. C. Moews, J. R. Knox, J. Frere, and J. Ghuysen, "Penicillin Target Enzyme and the Antibiotic Binding Site," *Science, 218,* 479–481 (1982).

37. "A New Wave of Antibiotics Builds," *Science, 214,* 1275–1278 (1981).

38. Demain, A. L., J. Kupa, Y.-Q. Shen, and S. Wolfe, "Microbial Synthesis of -Lactam Antibiotics," MIT Report 2-21-83 (1983).

39. Demain, A. L., "Regulation of -Lactam Antibiotic Production," MIT Report, 4-20-83 (1983).

40. Demain, A. L., "Formation of -Lactam Antibiotics by Microorganisms," MIT Report 4-19-83 (1983).

41. DeTilly, G., D. G. Mou, and C. L. Cooney, "Optimization and Economics of Antibiotic Production," MIT Report, 3-11-83 (1983).

42. Atkinson, B. and F. Matvituna. *Biochemical Engineering and Biotechnology Handbook.* The Nature Press (1982).

43. Baglioni, C. and T. W. Nielsen, "The Action of Interferon at the Molecular Level," *American Scientist, 69,* 392–399 (1981).

44. Marx, J. L., "Interferon (I): On the Threshold of Clinical Application," *Science, 204,* 1283–1286 (1979).

45. Marx, J. L., "Interferon (II): Learning About How it Works," *Science, 204,* 1293–1299 (1979).

46. Cantell, K., "Towards the Clinical Use of Interferon," *Chemtech,* 537–541 (Sept. 1979).

47. Blackwell, F., "Interferon: A Progress Report," *New Scientist, 29,* 783–785 (March 1982).

48. "Interferon Activity Without the Interferon," *Science, 219,* 292 (1983).

49. Lerner, T. J., "Interferon," *GEN,* 16 (Jan/Feb 1982).

50. Kramer, N., "Companies Producing Interferon: Who's Doing What?" *GEN,* 17–19 (Jan/Feb 1982).

51. Fix, J. L., "Tour de Force Yields Interferon in Bacteria," *C&EN,* 37–38 (Jan. 28, 1980).

52. Krananikas, M., "Interferon Synthesis: Yeast Emerges as Production Source Organism of Choice," *GEN,* 7 (Sept/Oct 1982).

53. "Gene Feat Spurs Interferon Race," *Chemical Week,* 43–44 (Feb. 6, 1980).

54. "Searle Building Interferon Plant," *Chemical Week,* 72 (March 12, 1980).

55. Cole, H. H. and M. Ronning, eds. *Animal Agriculture.* N. H. Freedman & Co., San Francisco (1974).

56. Parsons, J. A. *Peptide Hormones.* University Park Press, Baltimore (1976).

57. "Rushing with Synthetic Insulins," *Chemical Week,* 13 (March 2, 1983).

58. *Chemical Engineering,* 9 (Sept. 19, 1983).

59. Posner, M., "Polypeptide Hormones from Tissue Culture," in *Enzyme Engineering,* Vol. 2, E. K. Pye and L. B. Wingard, eds., Plenum Press, NY (1973).

60. Office of Technology Assessment, "Biotechnology: Commercialization and Internal Competitiveness," U.S. Congress, OTA (1983).

61. Robbins, K. C., H. N. Antoniades, S. G. Devare, M. W. Honkapiller, and S. A. Aaronson, 'Structural and Immunological Similarities Between Simian Sarcoma Virus Gene Product(s) and Human Platelet-Derived Growth Factor," *Nature, 305,* 605–608 (1983).

62. Devel, T. E., J. S. Huang, S. S. Huang, P. Stacobant, and M. D. Waterfield, "Expression of a Platelet-Derived Growth Factor Like Protein in Simian Sarcoma Virus Transformed Cells," *Science, 221,* 1348–1350 (1983).

63. Ibbotson, K. J., S. M. Disouza, K. W. Ng, C. K. Osborne, M. Niall, T. J. Martin, and C. R. Mundy, "Tumor-Derived Growth Factor Increases Bone Resorption in a Tumor Associated with Humoral Hypercalcemia of Malignancy," *Science, 221,* 1291–1294 (1983).

64. Sporn, M. B., A. B. Roberts, J. H. Shull, K. M. Smith, J. M. Ward, and A. J. Sodek, "Polypeptides Transforming Growth Factors Isolated from Bovine Sources and Used for Wound Healing in vivo," *Science, 219,* 1329–1331 (1983).

65. Barnes, D. W., J. Silnutzer, C. See, and M. Shaffer, "Characterization of Human Serum Spreading Factor with Monoclonal Antibody," *Proc. Natl. Acad. Sci., 80,* 1362–1366 (1983).

66. "Industrial Production of a Human Growth Factor," *Chemical Week,* 44 (Oct. 12, 1983).

67. *Genetic Technology News,* 5 (June 1983).

68. "Human T-Cell Growth Factor (Interleukin-2)," Company Brochure, Cellular Products Inc. (1983).

69. "Virus Made Protein Acts Like Growth Factor," *C&EN,* 18 (Sept. 28, 1983).

70. Schwick, H.-G. and H. Haupt, "Chemistry and Function of Human Plasma Proteins," *Angew. Chem. Int. E. Eng., 19,* 87–99 (1980).

71. Fraser, H. M., "A New Class of Contraceptives," *Nature, 296,* 391–392 (1982).

72. Newmark, P., *New Routes to Polypeptide," Nature, 280,* 637–678 (1979).

73. Chang, T. M. S., "Use of Immobilized Enzymes in Medical Practice," in *Enzymes,* J. P. Danehy and B. Wolnak, eds., Marcel Dekker, Inc., New York (1980).

74. Terminielio, L. and A. Lesuk, "Status and Potential for Enzymes as Parenteral Therapeutic Agents," in *Enzymes,* J. P. Danehy and B. Wolnak, eds., Marcel Dekker, Inc., New York (1980).

75. "Glutaminase Aids Anticancer Therapy in Animals," *CE&N,* 49 (Sept. 12, 1983).

76. Chang, T. M. S., "Use of Immobilized Enzymes in Medical Practice," in *Enzymes—The Interface Between Technology and Economics,* J. P. Danehy and B. Wolnak, eds., Marcel Dekker, Inc. (1980).

77. Langer, R. J., S. Hoffberg, A. K. Larsen, C. L. Cooney, D. Tapper, and M. Klein, "An Enzymatic System for Removing Heparin in Extracorporeal Therapy," *Science, 217,* 201–203 (1982).

78. Sherry, J., "Fibrinolygic Agent," *Disease of the Month,* Your Book Medical Publishers, Inc., Chicago (May 1969).

79. Bergmann, S. R., K. B. A. Fox, M. M. Ter-Pugossian, B. E. Sobel, and D. Collen, "Clot-Selective Coronary Thrombolysis with Tissue Type Plasminogen Activator," *Science, 220,* 1181–1183 (1983).

80. Anderson, J. L., H. W. Marshall, B. E. Bray, J. R. Lutz, P. R. Frederick, F. G. Yanowitz, F. L. Datz, S. C. Klausner, and A. D. Hagan, "A Randomized Trial of Intracoronary Streptokinase in the Treatment of Acute Myocardial Infarction," *New England Jnl. of Medicine, 308* (22), 1312–1318 (1983).

81. Khaja, F., J. A. Walton, Jr., J. F. Brymer, E. Lo, L. Osterberger, W. W. O'Neill, H. T. Colfer, R. Weiss, T. Lee, T. Kurian, A. D. Goldberg, B. Pitt, and S. Goldstein, "Intracoronary Fibronolytic Therapy in Acute Myocardial Infarction," *New England Jnl. of Medicine, 308* (22), 1305–1311 (1983).

82. Gronow, M. and R. Bliem, "Production of Human Plasminogen Activators by Cell Culture," *Trends in Biotechnology, 1* (1) (1983).

83. Venkatasubramanian, K., W. R. Vieth, and F. R. Bernath, "Use of Collagen Immobilized Enzymes in Blood Treatment," in *Enzyme Engineering, Vol. 2,* E. K. Pye and L. P. Wingard, eds., Plenum Press (1975).

84. "Enzyme Inducers for Diabetes," *New Scientist,* 15 (Oct. 6, 1983).

85. Prescott, L. M., "Firm Synthesizing Therapeutic Oligonucleotides Which Selectively Inhibit Translation in Viruses," *GEN,* 18–19 (Sept/Oct 1983).

86. Walsh, C. J., "Suicide Substrates: Mechanism-Based Inactivators of Specific Target Enzymes," MIT Advances in Applied Enzymology (May 10, 1983).

87. "Liver Cells Persuaded to Make Insulin," *New Scientist, 1,* 622 (Sept. 1983).

88. "Gene Injected into Deficient Cells," *C&EN,* 6 (Oct. 15, 1977).

89. "A New Route to Gene Therapy in Hereditary Disease," *New Scientist, 6,* 355 (May 1982).

90. Powledge, T. M., "Gene Therapy: Will It Work," *Technology Review,* 82–87 (Apr. 1983).

91. Baldwin, R. W., "Monoclonal Antibodies in the Diagnosis, Detection and Therapy of Cancer," *Proc. Royal Soc. of Edinburgh, 81B,* 261–276 (1982).

92. Vietta, E. S., W. Cushley, and J. W. Uhr, "Synergy of Ricin A Chain-Containing Immunotoxins and Ricin B Chain-Containing Immunotoxins in in vitro Killing of Neoplasal Human B Cells," *Proc. Natl. Acad. Sci., 80,* 6332–6335 (1983).

93. Weinstein, J. N., M. A. Steller, A. M. Keenan, D. G. Covelc, M. E. Key, S. M. Sieber, R. K. Oldham, K. M. Huang, and R. J. Parker, "Monoclonal Antibodies in the Lymphatic: Selective Delivery to Lymph Node Metastates of a Solid Tumor," *Science, 282,* 423–426 (1983).

94. Steplewski, Z., M. D. Lubeck, and H. Koprowski, "Human Macrophages Armed with Murine Immunoglobulin G2a Antibodies to Tumors Destroy Human Cancer Cells," *Science, 221,* 865–867 (1983).

95. Heath, T. D., J. A. Montgomery, J. R. Piper, and D. Papahadjopoulos, "Antibody-Targeted Liposomes: Increase in Specific Toxicity of Methotrexate--Aspartate," *Proc. Natl. Acad. Sci., 80,* 1377–1381 (1983).

96. Martinis, J. and C. Hill, " 'Bifunctional' Antibody Allows Specific Targeting of Anti-Tumor Agents," *GEN,* 38 (Sept/Oct 1982).

97. Solomon, S., "New Weapon Against Disease," *Science Digest,* 42–44 (Dec. 1983).

98. "Monoclonal Antibodies May Aid Victims of Brown Recluse Spider's Bite," *GEN,* 30 (March/April 1983).

99. Lerner, T. J., "Monoclonals Reverse Kidney Rejection," *GEN,* 3 (Sept/Oct 1981).

100. Waldor, M., S. Sriram, H. O. McDevitt, and L. Steinman, "In vivo Therapy with Monoclonal Anti-I-A Antibody Suppresses Immune Responses to Acetylcholine Receptor," *Proc. Natl. Acad. Sci., 80,* 2713–2717 (1983).

101. Dixon, B., "The New Shepherds of St. Kilda," *Science,* 52–55 (Sept. 1983).

102. Broun, G., "Trends in the Use of Immobilized Enzymes and Proteins in Human Therapeutics," in *Enzyme Engineering, Vol. 2,* E. K. Pye and L. B. Wingard, eds., Plenum Press (1975).

103. Chang, T. M. S., "Effects of Different Routes of *in vivo* Administration of Microencapsulated Enzymes," in *Enzyme Engineering,* Vol. 2, E. K. Pye and L. B. Wingard, eds., Plenum Press (1975).

104. Hersh, L. S., "*L. Asparaginase* from *Escherichia coli II* and *Erwinia Carotovura* Bound to Poly (methyl methacrylate)," in *Enzyme Engineering,* Vol. 2, E. K. Pye and L. B. Wingard, eds., Plenum Press (1975).

105. Cheremisinoff, P. N. and R. P. Ouellette, eds. *Biotechnology: Applications and Research.* Technomic Publishing Co., Inc., Lancaster, PA; Basel, Switz. (1985).

8

Biotechnology and Energy

INTRODUCTION

B *iotechnology plays today* only a minor role in energy prospection, extraction, conversion and utilization. The future potential is great in several specialized areas. Figure 8-1 presents the energy cycle in its simplest form. A number of biotechnology methods are applicable to each step in the cycle.

This chapter will review the state of the art of applying biotechnologies to the energy system with emphasis on fuels desulfurization, enhanced oil recovery, hydrogen production, energy and chemicals production from biomass and biological fuel cells.

MICROBIAL PROSPECTING

With rapid advances in industrial microbiology, the old method of geomicrobiological prospecting might be due for a renewal [1,2]. It is naive to believe that the existence of large energy reservoirs (coal, oil, gas), deep in the ground, would not affect the flora and fauna inhabiting the soil above. In that respect, microorganisms may be most important. Some 25–200 million microbes can be found in each gram in the upper layers of soil. Such organisms are well adapted to their environment and display great versatility as to their sources of energy and carbon. Certain obligate species have adapted to very special sources to supply their needs.

It is assumed that energy reservoirs would release chemical species affecting the balance of microorganisms in the immediate environment.

137

THE ENERGY CYCLE

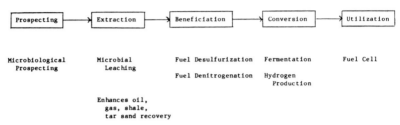

Figure 8-1. Applicability of biotechnology to energy.

This effect is blurred by a variety of other environmental effects. It is proposed that a spectrum of microorganisms might indicate the presence of potential reservoirs. The concept has been tested with promising results.

FUEL DESULFURIZATION

Some 50% of the U.S. electrical capacity is based on coal. We have extensive reserve of this energy source and no cartel exists to control its price. On the other hand, most of the U.S. coal contains sulfur and stringent environmental regulations preclude its use without pre-combustion, combustion or post-combustion control of its gaseous emission. Pre-combustion cleaning includes coal cleaning, gasification and liquefaction. Post-combustion takes the form of gas scrubbing. These techniques are relatively costly, adding some $20.00 to the cost of each ton of coal. The bacteria *Thiobacillus* and *Sulfolobus* provides a promising alternative.

Sulfur in coal is in three forms: 1) organic sulfur where the sulfur is covalently bonded to carbon or bound as a sulfate, 2) Pyritic sulfur in the form of pyrite and marcasite, and 3) sulfate. The percentage of sulfate is always less than 0.1 percent. The total sulfur content of U.S. coal ranges from about 0.25% to 7.0%. Generally, in coal containing more than 1% total sulfur, the percent of pyrite sulfur exceeds the content of organic sulfur [3].

The chemistry of coal desulfurization is as follows [4].

The bacillus (*T. ferrooxidans*) catalyzes the oxidation of pyrite.

$$2FeS_2 + 7.5\% + H_2O \xrightarrow{\text{Bacteria}} Fe_2(SO_4)_3 + H_2SO_4 \qquad (1)$$

The ferric sulfate produced by this reaction tends to hydrolyze and yield insoluble hydroxide and basic sulfates.

$$Fe_2(SO_4)_3 + 6H_2O \rightarrow 2Fe(OH)_3 + 3H_2SO_4 \qquad (2)$$

$$Fe_2(SO_4)_3 + 6H_2O \rightarrow 2Fe(OH)SO_4 + H_2SO_4 \qquad (3)$$

$$1.5\ Fe_2(SO_4)_3 + 6H_2O \rightarrow [H(Fe(SO_4)_2 \cdot Fe(OH)_3)] + 2.5\ H_2SO_4 \quad (4)$$

These reactions all contribute to the acidity of the milieu.
The ferric iron produced in reaction (1) can further oxidize the pyrite and other metal sulphides.

$$FeS_2 + 4\ Fe^{3+} \rightarrow 5\ Fe^{2+} + 2S^{\circ} \qquad (5)$$

$$MS + Fe^{3+} \rightarrow M^{+2} + 2\ Fe^{2+} + S^{\circ} \qquad (6)$$

The ferrous iron and the elemental sulfur are oxidized by the bacteria; respectively regenerating the oxidizing agent and contributing to acid production.

$$Fe^{2+} \xrightarrow{\text{T. ferrooxidans}} Fe^{3+} + e^- \qquad (7)$$

$$S^{\circ} + 1.5O_2 + H_2O \xrightarrow{\text{T. ferrooxidans}} H_2SO_4 \qquad (8)$$

Metal sulfide can also be oxidized directly by the bacteria.

$$MS + 2O_2 \xrightarrow{\text{T. ferrooxidans}} MSO_4 \qquad (9)$$

A recent quantitative study [4] on the oxidation of FeS_2 and pyrite in coal indicates a maximum rate of oxidation (V_m) of 25.1 to 66.5 mg/l/h for coal and 138.9 for FeS_2 and a value of the Michaelis-Menten factor (K_m) of 22.2 for FeS_2 and of 14.6 to 31.0 for coal (expressed in percent pulp density). The same study gives Q_{10} values in the range of 1.75 to 2.0 (in the 25-30 °C range); and activation energy (based on an Arrhenius plot) ranging from -38.8 to -44.3 KJ/mol).

Recent tests with *Thiobacillus ferrooxidans* and *Thiobacillus thiooxidans* indicate a 90% removal of pyrite sulfur in two weeks on coal smaller than 100 mesh [5]. The tests indicate optimum desulfurization at a pH of 2.5 and a temperature of 25 °C [6]. A cell concentration of 10^{11} cells per gram of fresh coal gave good results. Since the bacterial attack is really a surface phenomena, the exposed pyrite area is the main rate determining criterion. The rate of desulfurization is inversely proportional to the particle size.

For certain coals in a 20% slurry, some inhibition of the *Thiobacillus ferrooxidans* takes place attributed to organic compounds leached from the coal. When heterotrophic organisms (*T. perometabolis, T. acidephilus, T. novellus* and *T. neopolitanus*) are added to the slurry, they rapidly metabolize the organic compounds detrimental to the activity of *Thiobacillus ferrooxidans* and restore its full activity.

When similar tests were conducted with *Sulfolobus acidocaldarius* and related thermophilic organisms at 60 to 80 °C, the same results were obtained except that the 90% pyrite removal was achieved in six days [6].

An economic analysis based on an 8,000 ton per day coal facility and using lined and covered lagoons as reactors was conducted. Based on input coal with 2% sulfur, an 18-day residence time for 90% pyrite removal, a 99% coal recovery, a slurry at 20% of −200 mesh coal and a dewatering to 10% final moisture in the cleaned coal; the unit cost was $11.46/ton 1977 dollars [6].

The obvious advantages of the microbial leaching technique are lower cost and no reduction in the coal's heating value. The disadvantages include: 1) a long residence time 6–20 days. This is not such a problem if the cleaning system is in the 90-day onsite coal storage cycle of most electric utilities. 2) The need to grind the coal to a fine mesh. Here again, the coal is pulverized prior to feeding to modern coal burners. 3) The corrosion of the acidic environment requiring expensive corrosin-proof reactors. This can be alleviated by using lined and covered ponds. 4) The water content of the coal and the cost of dewatering. This problem can be eliminated if the microbial coal leaching process is for input to a coal-water or coal-alcohol slurry combustion system.

Scientists have isolated pseudomona-like microorganisms capable of converting sulfur and nitrogen containing aromatic compounds in liquid fossil fuels to water soluble species. Dibenzothiophenes and related compounds represent some 70% of the total organic sulfur in some Texas oils, in various vacuum oils and other high-boiling petroleum fractions. One group of organisms produce leucine which induces other organisms to oxidize dibenzothiophenes to water soluble products.

ENHANCED OIL RECOVERY

Enhanced oil recovery is a chemical flooding of producer wells. The method involves the injection of chemicals (polymers and surfactants) into an oil formation, to loosen up the oil and push it to producing wells. Polymers and surfactants are commercially produced by a number of chemical companies. The need arises to inject microorganisms, capable of producing the required chemicals, directly in the formation.

Exopolysaccharides are polysaccharides found outside the microbial cell wall and membrane and are a common product of microbial cells. Polysaccharides produced from microorganisms have advantages over those produced synthetically [7,8].

The one disadvantage is the high cost of installation and startup of fermentation equipment, together with large solvent requirements and the associated need for a considerable amount of energy. It appears that this disadvantage can be overcome given sufficient applciation, money and innovation.

The greatest single potential market for commercially produced exopolysaccharides is the oil industry. These polymers used in tertiary oil recovery improve water-flooding and micellar-polymer operations. The role of polymer is to reduce the flow capacity of the solution in the rock system. Xanthan, a bacterial exopolysaccharide from the genus *Xanthomones compestris*, has been shown to produce higher viscosity and low sensitivity to saline than the synthetic polymers. The effectiveness of an exopolysaccharide depends on the salinity, pH, temperature, viscosity and characteristics of an oil field. Currently, problems encountered in using Xanthan include plugging of the rock near wells due to the presence of particulate material (i.e., bacterial debris) and changes in the polysaccharide concentration due to chemical adsorption onto the permeable rock structure. Detailed research is underway to overcome these difficulties. Use of Xanthan as a drilling mud has been patented by Exxon [9].

Several important advances in enhanced oil recovery are worth reporting.

- A new biopolymer (trade name Emulsan) produced by *Acinetobacter calcoaceticus* appears promising for many surfactant uses: enhanced oil recovery, emulsifier for hydrocarbon water fuel mixtures, pipeline additives, etc. The polymer is lipoheteropolysaccharide to which fatty acid esters have been attached. The polysaccharide polymer is composed of galactosamine and aminouronic acid containing many hydrophilic groups. The lipophilic portion of the polymer is due primarily to the presence of 2- and 3-hydroxy dodecanoic acid esters. The molecular weight of the polymer is almost 1 million and the surface area occupied by the molecule is greater than 50,000 A^2 [10].
- A different glycolipid biopolymer produced by a bacterium belonging to the genus *Coryneform* can reduce the surface tension of crude oil-water mixtures to 2×10^{-2} dynes/cm—an effect compared to that of dodecyl sulfate—appears promising for EOR.

- Another genetically altered microorganism breaks down waxes and paraffins in heavy oils and produces CO_2 to further help oil recovery.
- In another case, *Zymonomas*, an anaerobic bacteria feeding on molasses, in situ, produces ethanol, higher alcohols, and organic acid with excellent surfactant properties.
- Another gene splitting effort aims at producing lipids and polypeptides with surfactant properties.

How to get water out of the oil is then a problem. Cultures of *Nocardia amarae* have shown an ability to de-emulsify both oil in water and water in oils emulsions. It is then possible to envisage a dual microbial system: one to emulsify the oil underground and the other one to de-emulsify the mixture upon its arrival at the surface.

Biotechnology also been applied to assist in a number of solid fuel extractions [11] (Table 8-1):

- coal processing to produce methane, other aliphatic hydrocarbons, and single cell protein;
- gas recovery from oil shale;
- oil extraction from shale;
- pretreatment of shale prior to retorting;
- extraction of hydrocarbons from tar sands;
- reduction of plugging and paraffin deposition in tar sands formations.

Present technology for production of oil from shale centers around a process of retorting. Retorting technology has some limitations:

1. Retorting requires an investment of thermal energy that must be subtracted from total energy production.
2. Retorting is inefficient, releasing about 50% of available hydrocarbons.
3. Formation of high-molecular-weight aromatic compounds inhibits refining efficiency, and they have been found to be carcinogenic.
4. Retorting results in large volumes of spent shale, which presents a disposal problem.

Bioleaching is an alternative shale technology that is currently under laboratory investigation. During bioleaching, sulfur-oxidizing bacterial species of the genus *Tiobacillus* (capable of producing sulfuric acid and ferric sulphate) are used. *Thiobacillus* in the presence of oil shale can use portions of the inorganic mineral matrix as a nutrient source. The acid medium produced by *Thiobacillus* has been shown to attack and chemically degrade the carbonate portion of the kerogen-entrapping inorganic mineral matrix. This develops porosity and permeability and increases the availability of internal surface in contact with the leaching medium.

TABLE 8-1. Summary of Applications of Biotechnology to Solid
Fossil Fuel Extraction/Processing.

Fossil Fuel	Application	Approach
Coal	Desulfurization	Use of microorganisms to remove inorganic sulfur from a coal slurry
		Heap leaching to remove sulfur
		Bacterial removal of organic sulfur
	Products from Coal	Methane from coal by the action of methanogenic bacteria
		Microbial production of aliphatic hydrocarbons using organisms indigenous to oil shale and other fossil fuel deposits
		Single cell protein from microorganisms grown on water extract of coal
Shale	Gas Recovery	Combination of chemical and bacterial treatment to release high and low BTu gases from black shale
	Oil Extraction	Microbial leaching of the inorganic matrix of oil shale/microbial breakdown of kerogen
		Microbial synthesis of aliphatic hydrocarbons from oil shale
	Pretreatment of Oil Shale	Bioleaching prior to retorting to remove sulfur and increase permeability
Tar Sands	Extraction of Hydrocarbons	Use of microbial surfactants to supplement solvent-surfactant cold water extraction
		Release of hydrocarbon residues from sands by contact with oxidase-synthesizing, hydrocarbon metabolizing microorganisms
		Use of bacteria to enhance solvent extractability and reduce sulfur and nitrogen content
	Reduction of Plugging and Paraffin Deposition in Tar Sand Deposits	Use of bacterial degradation of heavy hydrocarbons and paraffins to reduce plugging

Source: [11].

A continuous cyclic process has been developed that uses the bioleaching principle outlined above. Raw shale is continuously leached by gravity with a culture of *Thiobacillus thiooxidans*. The leachate is collected and supplemented with nutrients for growth of the sulfate reducer. The leached medium is innoculated with another autographic microbe, *Desulfovibro vulgaris*, and anaerobic conditions are initiated by a pyrogallic acid seal.

In Canada, mutated (by Radiation) strain of microorganisms cause formation of hydroxyl ions in tar, loosening it from the sand. The process operates at room temperature and yields 93% recovery of the tar from tar sands.

HYDROGEN PRODUCTION

Hydrogen production, based on sunlight energy and photosynthetic organisms, is depicted in Figure 8-2. The process is enzymatic in nature and makes use of hydrogenases and nitrogenases [12–23] (Figure 8-3).

A useful classification of organisms producing hydrogen is as follows:

1. Anaerobic fermentative bacteria, typified by *Clostridium* spp. (strict anaerobes).
2. Formate-hydrogen-lyase-possessing bacteria such as *Escherichia coli* and other enteric bacteria (facultative anaerobes).
3. Nitrogen-fixing bacteria, possessing nitrogenase.

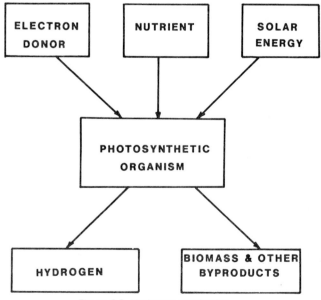

Figure 8-2. Hydrogen production.

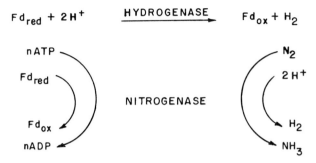

$$Fd_{red} + 2H^+ \xrightarrow{\text{HYDROGENASE}} Fd_{ox} + H_2$$

Figure 8-3. Hydrogen formation by biological systems. Source: [19].

4. Photosynthetic organisms:
   (a) photosynthetic bacteria (e.g., *Chromatium, Rhodopseudomonas*),
   (b) blue-green algae (cyanobacteria),
   (c) green algae (eukaryotes).

Biophotolysis is one of the approaches through which hydrogen, a nonpolluting fuel, could be produced by means of solar radiation. The most advanced system developed to date is based on the use of nitrogen-limited cultures of heterocystous blue-green algae.

In this system, H_2 and O_2 evolving reactions are separated at the microscopic level in the heterocysts and vegetative cells of these filamentous blue-green algae. Nitrogen-limited cultures of *Anabaena cylindrica* have been shown to evolve H_2 up to four weeks, both in the laboratory and outdoors.

The biophotolysis reaction gives a discontinuous production of H_2 because of the diurnal cycle. It has been demonstrated that H_2 production activities respond very rapidly to the start of sunshine in the morning, reaching a maximum within 30 minutes of direct sunlight on the converter. A similar reverse pattern is demonstrated at sunset. The limiting factors in H_2 production are the length of the algal filaments in the cultures, N_2-level and presence of reductant in the system.

Photosynthetic bacteria are known to produce energy in the form of hydrogen from an oxidizable organic source, but they are incapable of oxidizing water. Hence, no O_2 is evolved in bacterial photosynthesis. On the other hand, blue-green algae do produce O_2. In laboratory systems, the photosynthetic bacterium *Rhodospirillum rubrum* and the blue-green algae *Anacystis nidulans* are combined into a single system, with resultant production of H_2 plus O_2 by undergoing the following reaction [24]:

$$\text{A. nidulaus} \quad 2H_2O + 2NADP^+ \rightarrow O_2 + 2H^+ + 2NADPH$$

$$R.\ rubrum\ 2NADPH\ +\ 2H^+\ \rightarrow\ 2NADP\ +\ 2H_2O$$

Anacystis nidulens can produce NADPH from exogenously supplied NADP by the oxidation of water in a light reaction. This reduced NADPH can be reoxidized by *Rhodospirillum rubrum* to produce H_2.

A variety of algae (blue-green and purple) and bacteria produce hydrogen. Before this hydrogen can be used as a fuel source, it has to be separated from oxygen and other gases produced by these organisms. This is generally an energy-consuming process. The light-dependent production of hydrogen by photosynthetic bacteria offers a potential solution to this problem during this process, since CO_2 is the only additional gas evolved. Algae are known to use water as a hydrogen donor whereas purple nonsulfur bacteria require an organic substrate. It has been shown that a high yield of hydrogen can be achieved using lactic acid-containing cheese waste as both a hydrogen donor and carbon source for photosynthetic bacteria.

In laboratory systems, *Rhodospirillum rubrum* is the light-dependent photosynthetic bacterium that utilizes lactic acid waste substrates. The cultures are incubated anaerobically in a closed vessel at 30°C under continuous illumination. In laboratory experiments, production of H_2 of 65 ml/hr/L of culture volume is achieved. These results are comparable with the hydrogen production rates obtained with the blue-green alga *Anabaena*.

One potential method of producing energy in the form of hydrogen gas is to use microorganisms capable of oxidizing an organic compound in the presence of light. The bacterium known to do this is *Rhodospirillium rubrum*, a nonsulfur purple bacterium. The process outlined below uses immobilized *R. Rubrum* and malate as a substrate to produce H_2 in a continuous process. The reaction of this bioconversion is as follows [25]:

$$C_4H_6O_5(\text{Malate}) + 3H_2O \rightarrow 4CO_2 + 6H_2$$

Immobilization of *R. rubrum* is achieved by the following steps. A 4-g amount (wet weight) is added to 15 ml of Noble Agar 5% solution. This solution is spread evenly on both sides of a plastic slab composed of a series of thin plastic layers. The slab is then put into an airtight system. The system is immersed in water maintained at 18–19°C. The gas produced is channeled to a double-ended glass tube that is kept airtight by septums. The malate solution is pulled through the collector with a syringe, displacing any gas with substrate. Collection of the produced gas displaces the liquid. A sample is taken after the gas and the malate have equilibrated, and then a constant flowrate is reestablished.

Illumination for this process is provided by a rack of seven 100-Watt standard incandescent bulbs on each side of the reactor.

Based on this laboratory experiment, researchers feel that whole cells of *R. rubrum* can be immobilized in an active form in which they will produce H_2 on a continuous basis. Based on the 1976 dollar value, researchers suggest that this process is not economical at a cost of $10/lb of malate. This works out to a cost of $8.33/1000 ft^3. The heating capacity of H_2 is about one third that of natural gas vol/vol. Thus the price is equivalent to $25/1000 ft^3 natural gas based on raw materials (substrate) cost only.

ENERGY AND CHEMICALS FROM BIOMASS

The enzymatic conversion of cellulose waste to glucose is due to the action of cellulase from mutant fungus strains. The crude glucose is then used in a microbial fermentation process to produce alcohols, chemical feedstocks and single cell proteins.

Methane can be produced in anaerobic digester from manure and other biological waste material [26–28]. Algae can produce liquid hydrocarbons by reacting microscopal green plants with inexpensive hydrogen [29]. Ethanol, furfural, phenol, acetic acid, n-butanol, maleic anhydride, lignosulfonates, etc., are all possible products derived from biorefineries.

In the past, the enzymatic route has not progressed as rapidly as the chemical (acid hydrolysis) route. Recent progress in enzymology and fermentation will change this picture dramatically.

- The ability of *Pachysolen tannophilus* to convert pentoses (xylose) to ethanol and carbon dioxide (NRC Canada, USDA).
- The discovery that *Cyathus stercoreus* can break down lignin (USDA).
- The well demonstrated capability of *Trichoderma reesei* and *T. viridex* (Cleveland State U.) to break down cellulose.
- The observation that *Clostridium thermocellum* and *C. thermosaccharolyticum* can break down starches and ferment the sugar simultaneously (MIT).
- Progresses made in butanol fermentation using *Clostrium acatobutylicum* (Kansas State) and in ethanol production using *Zymomonas mobilis* (University of Queenland, Australia).
- New strains of *Candida* to ferment both glucose and xylose substrates (Purdue University).

• Recent advances in propionic/acetic acids production through the service of *Propionibacterium acidi-propionici* (University of Arkansas).
• The anaerobic bioconversion of one-carbon compounds (University of Wisconsin).
• Studies on the production of beta-hydroxypropionaldehyde via glycerol fermentation (USDA).

Recombinant DNA is being used to engineer better microorganisms. A variety of species are being studied as a source of crude oil. The eukaryotic alga *Botryococcus braunii* is such an organism. Crude oil content may reach 50% of dry weight. The crude oil contains a lipid and an hydrocarbon fraction. The hydrocarbons are C_{27} to C_{31} linear di-and tri-alpha-olefins. These are valuable feedstocks that could be craked to chemical feedstocks. The protein content of the cell may reach as high as 30%.

BIOLOGICAL FUEL CELLS

Fuel cells are devices which produce electricity and thermal energy directly from fuel and oxygen by electrochemical reactions. Fuel cells are most interesting because of their high thermal efficiency (46%), their ability to use liquid or gaseous hydrocarbons, their virtual lack of air pollution emission, and their modular nature.

A fuel cell consists basically of two thin porous plate electrodes separated by an electrolyte layer. A fuel gas stream containing a high proportion of hydrogen is catalytically converted into electrons and hydrogen ions at the negative electrode (anode). The ions move through the electrolyte while the electrons move through an external circuit (load). At the positive electrode (cathode), the ions and electrons combine with oxygen (from air) to produce water, at the same time releasing some heat.

Current fuel cells use phosphoric acid as the electrolyte; more advanced types now being researched will use molten carbonates or solid oxides as the electrolyte. The phosphoric acid fuel cell operates at about 400 °F (200 °C) with a net efficiency near 40%. Efficiencies of up to 46% are expected in the future from commercial systems. The advanced designs using different electrolytes will operate at higher temperatures, 1200–1800 °F, (650–1000 °C) and higher efficiencies. Since each cell is capable of only limited power output, fuel cells are combined into stacks to obtain the désired voltage and power output.

A number of fuel cell systems are under development and testing by private industries and under government sponsorship [30].

Phosphoric acid fuel cell
Solid polymer electrolyte fuel cell
Ammonia-fueled alkaline fuel cell
Trifluoromethane sulfuric acid fuel cell

Live microorganisms and purified enzymes have been used in biological fuel cells where oxidative degeneration reactions generate electrical energy. The key feature of such a system is the transfer of electron from the organism or enzyme to the anode [31–33]:

$$\begin{array}{c} \text{Microorganism} \\ \text{or Enzyme} \end{array} + \begin{array}{c} \text{mediator} \\ \text{(oxidized)} \end{array} \rightleftharpoons \begin{array}{c} \text{microrg} \\ \text{enzyme} \end{array} + \begin{array}{c} \text{mediator} \\ \text{(reduced)} \end{array}$$

$$\text{Mediator (oxidized)} \rightleftharpoons \text{mediator (reduced)} + 2H^+ + 2e^-$$

Any reaction involving oxidation (at the anode) and reduction (at the cathode) can be used in a fuel cell. Since a fuel cell operates on charge transfer rather than heat transfer, its efficiency is not subject to the Carnot cycle limitations. Hence high efficiency is possible. The slowness of electron transfer reactions at electrodes is a major problem.

A number of workable biological systems using microorganisms (e.g., *E. coli*) and enzymes (e.g., alkaline phosphatase, β-glucosidase, hydrogenases, cytochrome oxidases), in direct contact or incorporated into the electrodes have produced limited continuous currents over many days.

A methanol dehydrogenase biofuel cell generated 13.2 mA at 0.3V for a 10 ohm resistance with 5 mg of enzyme. Calculations from the experimental system indicate that a 6 M^3 gross volume cell would generate 1 kW of power [34].

CONCLUSION

Microbial and enzymatic systems are not yet major contributors to the energy cycle of the modern society.

Coal, oil, gas are concentrated forms of energy, rather inefficiently converted to heat. In spite of inefficiency and pollution problems, they will remain our major sources of energy until fusion and fission replace them. All other energy systems known to man either operate on a dilute source of energy, or with lower efficiency, or are usable only on a small case. In other words, they are a poor match to the large-scale, massive energy demanded by the industrial world. This does not mean that they have no role to play, only that their role will be different than the traditional systems.

Biological systems, fine tuned by the techniques of biotechnology, are likely to have major impacts on enhanced oil recovery and alcohol production. Other applications require major developments before competing in the marketplace.

REFERENCES

1. Serley, J. Q., "A Geomicrobiological Method of Prospecting for Petroleum, Part I," *The Oil & Gas Journal, 8,* 142-146 (April 1974).
2. Serley, J. Q., "A Geomicrobiological Method of Prospecting for Petroleum, Part 2," *The Oil & Gas Journal, 15,* 98-101 (April 1974).
3. Dungan, P. R. and W. A. Apel, "Microbial Desulfurization of Coal," in *Metallurgical Applications of Bacterial Leaching and Related Microbial Phenomena,* L. E. Murr, B. E. Thomas, and J. A. Brierly, eds., Academic Press (1978).
4. Olsen, T. M., P. R. Ashman, A. E. Torma, and L. E. Murr, "Desulfurization of Coal by *Thobacillus Ferrooxidans,*" in *Biogeochemistry of Ancient and Modern Environment,* P. A. Trudinger, M. R. Walter, and B. J. Ralph, eds., Springer-Verlag (1980).
5. Detz, C. M. and G. Barvinchak, "Microbial Desulfurization of Coal," *Mining Congress Journal,* 75-82 (July 1979).
6. Andrews, G. F. and J. Maczuga, *Bacterial Coal Desulfurization,* 4th Symposium for Biotechnology in Energy Production and Conservation, Gatlinburg, TN (1982).
7. Silman, R. W. and P. Rogovin, "Continuous Fermentation to Produce Xanthan Biopolymers: Laboratory Investigation," *Biotechnol. Bioeng., 12,* 75-83 (1970).
8. Yen, T. F., "Microbial Oil Shale Extraction," in *Microbial Energy Conversion,* Schlegel and Baruea, eds., Pergamon Press, Inc., Elmsford, NY (1977).
9. Sutherland, I. W. and D. C. Ellwood, "Microbial Exopolysaccharide Industrial Polymers of Current and Future Potential," in *Symposium Soc. for Generic Microbiology,* A. T. Bull, D. C. Ellwood, and C. Ratledge, eds., No. 29, Microbial Technology: Current State, Future Prospects, Cambridge Univ. Press (1979).
10. "New Biopolymer Vies for Many Surfactant Uses," *Chenical Engineering, 2,* 20-22 (May 1983).
11. Clerman, R. and R. Brown, "Survey of the Application of Biotechnologies to Solid Fossil for Extraction and Processing," The MITRE Corp., WP83W00253 (May 1983).
12. Mitsui, A., Y. Ohta, J. Frank, S. Kumazawa, C. Hill, D. Rosner, S. Barciella, J. Greenbaum, L. Haynes, L. Oliva, P. Dalton, J. Radway, and P. Giffard, "Photosynthetic Bacteria as Alternative Energy Sources: Overview of Hydrogen Production Resources," in *Alternative Energy Sources II, Volume 8, Hydrogen Energy,* T. N. Vezidoglu, ed., Hemisphere Publ. Co., Washington, D.C., pp. 3483-3510 (1980).
13. Greenbaum, E., "Application of Intact Algae to the Biophotolysis Problem," *Biotechnology and Bioengineering Symp. No. 12,* John Wiley & Sons, Inc. (1982).
14. Matsunaga, T. and A. Mitsui, "Seawater-Based Hydrogen Production by Immobilized Marine Photosynthetic Bacteria," *Biotechnology and Bioengineering Symp. No. 12,* John Wiley & Sons, Inc. (1982).

15. Ohta, Y., J. Frank, and A. Mitsui, "Hydrogen Production by Marine Photosynthetic Bacteria: Effect of Environmental Factors and Substrate Specificity on the Growth of a Hydrogen-Producing Marine Photosynthetic Bacterium, *Chromatium* Sp. Miami PBS 1071," *Int. J. Hydrogen Energy, 6* (5), 451–460 (1982).

16. Mitsui, A., "Saltwater Based Biological Solar Energy Conversion for Fuel, Chemicals, Fertilizer, Food and Feed," in *Proceedings of Bio-Energy 1980 World Congress and Exposition,* Bio-Energy Council, Washington, D.C. (1980).

17. Mitsui, A., E. Duerr, S. Kumazawa, E. Phlips, and H. Skjoldal, "Biological Solar Energy Conversion: Hydrogen Production and Nitrogen Fixation by Marine Blue-Green Algae," in *Sun II Proceedings of the International Solar Energy Society Silver Jubilee Congress,* Vol. I, K. W. Boer and B. H. Glenn, eds., Pergamon Press, pp. 31–35 (1979).

18. Kumazawa, S. and A. Mitsui, "Characterization and Optimization of Hydrogen Photoproduction by a Saltwater Blue Green Alga, *Oscillatoria* Sp. Miami Bg7.1. Enhancement Through Limiting the Supply of Nitrogen Nutrients," *Int. J. Hydrogen Energy, 6* (4), 341–350 (1981).

19. Smith, G. D., "Microbiological Hydrogen Formation," *Search, 9* (6), 209–213 (1978).

20. Mitsui, A., "Biological and Biochemical Hydrogen Production," in *Solar-Hydrogen Energy Systems,* T. Ohta, ed., Pergamon Press, pp. 171–191 (1979).

21. Mitsui, A., "Nitrogen and Hydrogen Metabolism in Marine Tropical Photosynthetic Protoryotes," 5th Intnl. Symposium on Photosynthetic Prokaryotes, Bombannes-Bordeau, France (1982).

22. Kumazawa, S. and A. Mitsui. *Hydrogen Metabolism of Photosynthetic Bacteria and Algae.* CRC Handbook of Biosolar Resources, Vol. 1, Part 1, CRC Press, Inc. (1982).

23. Ohta, Y. and A. Mitsui, "Enhancement of Hydrogen Production by Marine *Chromatium* Sp. Miami PBS 1071 Grown in Molecular Nitrogen," in *Advances in Biotechnology, Vol. II,* M. Moo-Young and C. W. Robinson, eds., pp. 303–307, Pergamon Press (1981).

24. Benemann, J. R., K. Miyamoto, and P. C. Hallenbeck, "Bioengineering Aspects of Biophotolysis," *Enzyme Microbiol. Technol., 2,* 103–111 (1980).

25. Miyamoto, K., P. C. Hallenbeck, and J. R. Benemann, "Solar Energy Conversion by Nitrogen-Limited Cultures of Anabaena Cylindrica," *J. Fermentation Technol., 57* (4), 287–293 (1979).

26. Coppinger, E., J. Brautigam, J. Lenart, and E. D. Baylon, "Report on the Design and Operation of a Full-Scale Anaerobic Dairy Manure Digester," SERI/FR-312-471 Prepared for DOE by Ecotope Group, Seattle, WA (1979).

27. Jewell, W. J., S. Dell'Orto, K. J. Fanfoni, T. D. Hayes, A. P. Leuschner, and D. F. Sherman, "Anaerobic Fermentation of Agricultural Residues: Potential for Improvement and Implementation—Final Report," Vol. II, Project No. DE-ACO2-76ET20051 (1980).

28. Fraser, M. D., "The Economics of SNG Production by Anaerobic Digestion of Specially Grown Plant Matter," in *Symposium Papers: Clean Fuels from Biomass on Wastes,* Sponsored by the Institute of Gas Technology, Washington, D.C., pp. 425–439 (1977).

29. "Oil from Algae: Blue Sky or Realistic Goal?" *Chem. Wk.,* 43–44 (July 18, 1979).

30. Roberts, R., "Status of the DOE Battery and Electrochemical Technology Program IV," The MITRE Corp., MTR 82W232 (May 1983).

31. Higgins, I., J. and H. Allen, and O. Hills, "Microbial Generation and Interconversion of Energy Sources," in *Symposium Soc. for Generic Microbiology,* A. T. Bull, D. C. Ellwood, and C. Ratledge, eds., No. 29, Microbial Technology: Current State, Future Prospects, Cambridge Univ. Press (1979).

32. Bennetto, H. P. and J. L. Stirling, "Anodic Reactions in Microbial Fuel Cells," *Biotechnology and Bioengineering, 25,* 559–568 (1983).

33. Razumas, V. I., Y. Y. Kulis, and A. A. Malinavskas, "Study of Alkaline Phosphatase and β-Glucosidase in an Electrochemical Cell," in *Microbial Enzyme Reactions Proceedings of the 5th Conf. of Project IV, Microbial Enzyme Reactions of the US/USSR Joint Working Group on the Production of Substances by Microbiological Methods,* PB-80-233803 (1980).

34. Turner, D. P., W. J. Aston, I. J. Higgins, G. Davis, and H. A. O. Hills, "Applied Aspects of Bioelectrochemistry: Fuel Cells, Sensors and Bioorganic Synthesis," *Biotechnology and Bioengineering Symp., 12,* 401–412 (1982).

9

Biotechnology and Environmental Protection

INTRODUCTION

The natural decomposition of inorganic and organic materials has occurred for millions of years. The biological management of waste has been practiced for thousands of years. Most microorganisms in use are extracted from soil and water bodies and use organic and toxic materials as sources of energy and carbon.

The practice in the past has been to use the microorganisms as found in soil and water or to artificially mutate these organisms to strains more effective in performing the task at hand.

While the future of biological treatment will be based on microorganisms; a drastic departure from the past will take place based on the new science of recombinant DNA.

This chapter is a broad overview of the accumulated experience in using microorganisms for waste treatments. Biodegradation of chemicals, sulfur and nitrogen compounds removal, and metal accumulation are emphasized.

BIODEGRADATION

A great deal of interest was created by Chakrabarty and his work on a "Superbug" while at General Electric. This is a case of cross-breeding rather than recombinant DNA [1]. Bacteria have the ability to pass plasmid back and forth between individuals of the same species and even between species. The technique used by Chakrabarty involves establishing a mixed colony of bacteria and exposing them to a chemical

153

stress. By repeating this process, he eventually bred a strain containing four different oil degrading plasmids [2].

Microbiologists have been feverishly active since, as can be seen from the following examples taken from the recent literature (see also Table 9-1).

- Some 20 different bacteria are said to be capable of breaking down polychlorinated biphenyls into water and carbon dioxide. One of these organisms from the genus *Alcaligenes* is photoactivated by sunlight. Sunlight enhances the speed of degradation of PCB by some 400% [3].
- Researchers, involved in training bacteria—*Bacillus megaterium* and *Nocardiopsis* to consume dioxin, observe that dioxin could more easily

TABLE 9-1. Microbial Degradation of Various Organic Pollutants.

Pollutant	Microbes involved
I. Petroleum hydrocarbons	200+ species of bacteria, yeasts, and fungi; e.g., *Acinetobacter, Arthrobacter, Mycobacteria, Actinomycetes,* and *Pseudomonas* among bacteria; *Cladosporium* and *Scolecobasidium* among yeasts
II. Pesticides/herbicides cyclodiene type (e.g., aldrin, dieldrin)	*Zylerion xylestrix* (fungus)
organophosphorus type (e.g., parathion, malathion)	*Pseudomonas*
2,4-D	*Pseudomonas, Arthrobacter*
DDT	*Penicillium* (fungus)
kepone	*Pseudomonas*
piperonylic acid	*Pseudomonas*
III. Other chemicals	
bis (2-ethylhexyl)phthalate	*Serratia marascens* (bacteria)
dimethylnitrosamine	photosynthetic bacteria
ethylbenzene	*Nocardia tartaricans* (bacteria)
pentachlorophenol	*Pseudomonas*
IV. Lignocellulosic wastes	
municipal sewage	*Pseudomonas* *Thermonospora* (a thermophilic bacterium)
pulp mill lignins (various phenols)	yeasts: *Aspergillus* *Trichosporon* bacteria: *Arthrobacter* *Chromobacter* *Pseudomonas* *Xanthomonas*

Source: [10]

penetrate the cell walls and be degraded faster if solvents such as ethyl acetate and dimethyl sulfoxide were added to the broth [4].

- A strain of genetically engineered microorganisms degrades 95% or more of the persistent 2,4,5,T within a week. Microbes can also degrade a variety of dichlorobiphenyls and chlorobenzoates [5].

- Scientists have isolated a strain of *Pseudomonas* that uses 2,4,D as a source of carbon. The gene involved was isolated and inserted in a different host bacteria [6].

- A number of microorganisms containing plasmids bearing genes for the degradation of aromatic molecules—toluene and xylene (TOL), diverse salicylates (SAL) and chloride derivatives of 4-chlorocatecol (pAC 25) have been tested [7].

- Formulation of bacterial mutants are commercially available for a variety of wastewater treatment problems. Specially formulated preparations are used for petroleum refinery/petroleum chemical plant wastewaters cleanup. The bacteria degrade various hydrocarbons and organic chemicals (benzenes, phenols, cresols, naphthalenes, amines, alcohols, synthetic detergents, petroleum (crude and processed)) [8].

- Grease eating bacteria have successfully been used in cleaning clogged sewers [9].

- A major problem in recent decades has been the appearance of new chemicals in the environment stretching the ability of microorganisms to evolve by adaptation of existing catabolic enzymes or by the appearance of new metabolic pathways, the ability to degrade persistent xenobiotic compounds. Man is constantly learning from such organisms and is selecting those that show a maximum rate of biodegradation with maximum substrate utilization and minimum microbial biomass production [11].

DESULFURIZATION

The bacteria, expert at mineral leaching, can be applied to water decontamination in conjunction with other microorganisms.

In many mining operations, water is pumped out of the mines to prevent flooding. Water used in milling processes becomes laden with soluble inorganic ions. Mine drainage from abandoned mines is loaded with a variety of metal salts. The practice has been to evaporate this water in holding ponds or to neutralize the acid flow and precipitate the metals with lime.

Many organisms have the ability to concentrate, accumulate or precipitate metals allowing the recovery of elements of economic importance. Many bacteria are known to concentrate potassium, magnesium, manganese, iron, calcium, nickel and cobalt. Other bacteria produce complexing agents which selectively extract metals from dilute solutions. Algaes concentrate silica, green-brown algae and fungi concentrate zinc and other heavy metals. Mosses and higher plants concentrate mercury, nickel, zinc, uranium, cesium and strontium.

Sulfite reducing bacteria of the *Desulfovibrio, Desulfotomaculum, Desulfobacter, Desulfococcus, Desulfonema,* and *Desulfosarcina* genera are especially adept at metal removal from water by producing hydrogen sulfide which precipitate these metals [12]. The constituent members of these groups embrace a wide range of salinity or osmotic pressure, temperature, hydrostatic pressure, pH, Eh, and other environmental conditions [13].

These organisms have been put to work in mine wastewater cleanup operations [14]. In a real case, settling ponds innoculated with sulfate reducing bacteria (*Desulfovibrio, Desulfotomaculum*), and sulfur oxidizing thiobacilli (*Thiobacillus thiooxidans, T. thiopiaus, T. denitrificans*), and algae (*Chara, Spirogyra, Oscillatoria*) have been effective in lowering the concentration of uranium, selenium, and molybdenum in wastewater.

A variety of metallurgical effluents containing high concentrations of sulfate ions. A number of microorganisms can utilize this sulfate and convert it to an insoluble, stable, non-leachable form. *Desulfovibrio* reduces sulfate to sulfide. *Chlorobium* and *Chromatium* photosynthetically oxidize sulfide to elemental sulfur. A mutuallism between these bacteria was proposed [15].

$$SO_4^{=} \xrightarrow{\text{Desulfovibrio}} H_2S \xrightarrow[\text{Chromatium}]{\text{Chlorobium or}} S^{\circ}$$

A series of tests applied to solvent extraction raffinate demonstrates that a gas purged mutuallistic system of *Desulfovibrio* and *Chlorobium* can be used for the efficient conversion of sulfate to elemental sulfur.

The depletion of high grade ore parallel the exponentially increasing demand for metals to support the industrialized world. The extraction of minerals from ores, its beneficiation to a high quantity material, and its fabrication into a useful product are all sources of very toxic materials. Many industrial wastes contain valuable metals diluted in a large mass or volume. Processes must be developed to simultaneously extract these valuable metals and reduce the attack on our environment.

A series of tests have been conducted using *T. ferrooxidans* and *T. thiooxidans* to extract economically interesting metals from wastes: 1) jarosite—a residue which accumulates during zinc production; 2) sulidic dust concentrates from copper processing; 3) fly ash from a pyrite-roasting process; 4) slag from a lead smelting process [16]. The results indicate that it is possible to stimulate bacteria already at work on these waste dumps to leach into solution economically valuable metals.

Flotation is probably the most common unit operation in metallurgical operations. One of the problems is that the reject water is laden with flotation chemical agents. Recent laboratory experiments have tested the ability of *Escherichia coli, Proteus rettgerii, Klebsiella pneumoniae* and *Pseudomonas aerucinosa* to biodegrade sodium hexadecylsulfate, sodium oleate and dodecylamine acetate [17]. *Klebsiella* and *Proteus* appear to be the most efficient organisms. They handled very well the sodium hexadecyl sulfate, manage with the sodium oleate but had difficulty with the amine. *Pseudomonas fluoresccens* has been used to remove flotation agents from wastewaters [18].

NITRIFICATION/DENITRIFICATION

The nitrogen cycle is complex like all biogeological cycles. Its essential components are:

1) Nitrogen fixation

$$N_2 + H^+ \xrightarrow{\text{Rhizobium}} NH_3$$

2) Nitrification

$$NH_3 + O_2 \xrightarrow{\text{Nitrosomas}} NO_2^-$$

$$NO_2^- + O_2 \xrightarrow{\text{Nitrobacter}} NO_3^=$$

3) Denitrification

$$NH_3 + NO_3^= \xrightarrow{\text{Pseudomonas}} H_2O \text{ or } N_2$$

During biological denitrification, bacteria reduce nitrite or nitrate to nitrogen gas. The heterotrophic bacteria require a source of carbon. In denitrification reactions, this supplemental source is often provided by methanol. The nitrogen reaction is a respiratory process encompassing the following reactions [19].

$$NO_3 + 1/3 \ CH_3OH \rightarrow NO_2 + CO_2 + 2/3 \ H_2O$$

$$\underline{NO_2 + 1/2 \ CH_3CH \rightarrow 1/2 \ N_2 + 1/2 \ CO_2 + 1/2 \ H_2O + OH}$$
$$NO_3 + 5/6 \ CH_3OH \rightarrow 1/2 \ N_2 + 5/6 \ CO_2 + 7/8 \ H_2O + OH$$

Biological reactions have been used in the conversion of ammonia-nitrogen to nitrate-nitrogen with attendant reduction in chemical oxygen demand and total organic carbon [20,21] in coal gasifier effluents and municipal wastewaters.

WASTEWATER TREATMENT

Most biological wastewater treatment processes use aerobic reactors with its attendant large energy costs for aeration. Recently, a number of groups have turned to anaerobic bioreactors for either municipal wastewater treatment [22,23], or for specialized industrial wastewater treatment systems [20,24]. Engineering up to the pilot scale level indicates substantial energy and cost savings by comparison with traditional systems.

A number of enzymes have been applied to wastewater cleanups. A dramatic case is the use of horseradish peroxidase and hydrogen peroxide for the removal of phenol from coal conversion aqueous effluents [25]. Ninety-seven to 99% phenol removal was achieved over a wide range of pH and phenol concentration.

METAL CONCENTRATION AND REMOVAL

Metal ions, especially heavy metals, are highly toxic to microorganisms. Over the years these organisms have evolved a variety of defense mechanisms to cope with this threat. Four mechanisms are important [26].

1. Reduction to Free Metals

Various bacteria play a role in converting metallic salts to the metal form. Mercury is the metal best studied. The gene specifying the enzymes for this conversion has been shown to be plasmid-born. More than 200 such plasmids have been characterized in enteric bacteria such as *Staphylococcus aureus* and *Pseudomonas*.

2. Minimization of Metal Uptake

The resistance to certain metals (e.g., resistance against Cd^{+2} in *Staphylococcus aureus*) is achieved by changes in the permeability of the membrane for the metal. This resistance factor is also carried on a plasmid.

3. Concentration of Metal Intracellularly

A number of bacteria can store metals intracellularly in an inactivated form. Binding to a protein is a preferred method. This detoxification method has been demonstrated for mercury, cadmium, arsenic, lead and zinc in *S. aureus*; and for mercury in *Enterobacter aerogenes* and *Pseudomonas* strains.

4. Methylation of Metals

A number of organisms harbor a plasmid allowing them to methylate metals. Since most methylated metals are volatile, this represents an effective detoxication and resistance mechanism. This has been shown for mercury in *Pseudomonas* strains.

The astute scientist can take advantage of the work of evolution in utilizing such specialized microorganisms for toxic metal concentration, sequestration and removal.

CONCLUSION

The "High Tech" side of biotechnology has not yet penetrated the environmental protection market. Not a lack of interest or challenging problem, but a soft and diffuse marketplace is responsible.

It is expected that over the next few years the random approach of organisms isolation-mutation-selection will be systematically replaced by the more fine-tuned recombinant DNA technique to engineer organisms capable of detoxifying air, water, soil and waste materials.

The field of environmental monitoring would also gain by marrying biotechnology to the existing detection hardware taking the pulse of our environment. The general emphasis on toxic chemicals in their associated diversity will do much to speed up this process. Already, enzymatic systems are creating themselves a niche as reagent for environmental monitoring. The next step cannot be far behind.

REFERENCES

1. "Building 'Superbugs' for the Big Cleanup," *Chemical Week, 83,* 39 (June 1980).
2. "Bacteria Combat Waste," *Genetic Engineering News,* 9 (May/June 1981).
3. *Inside R&D, 1983,* 5 (March 1982).
4. *Chemical Week,* 29 (June 29, 1983).
5. *Inside R&D,* 1 (July 8, 1981).
6. *Inside R&D,* 1 (July 9, 1980).
7. "Les Microbes contre la Pollution Chemique," *La Recherche, 131,* 382–383 (1982).
8. Tracy, K. D. and T. G. Zitrides, "Mutant Bacteria Aids Exxon Waste System," *Hydrocarbon Proc.* (Oct. 1979).
9. Baig, N. and E. M. Grenning, "The Use of Bacteria to Reduce Clogging of Sewer Lines by Grease in Municipal Sewage," in *Biological Control of Water Pollution,* Tourbeir and Pierson, eds., University of Pennsylvania Press, Philadelphia, 245–252 (1976).
10. Zaugg, R. H. and J. R. Swarz, "Assessment of Future Environmental Trends and Problems: Industrial Use of Applied Genetics and Biotechnology," PB 82-118911 (1981).
11. Slater, J. H. and H. J. Somerville, "Microbial Aspects of Waste Treatment with Particular Attention to the Degradation of Organic Compounds," in *Microbial Technology: Current State, Future Prospects,* 29th Symposium, Society for General Microbiology, Cambridge, Cambridge Univ. Press (1979).
12. Peck, H. D. and L. G. Ljungdahl, "The Microbiology and Physiology of Anaerobic Fermentation of Cellulose," DOE/ER/10499-2, DE82 015522 (1982).
13. ZoBell, C. E., "Ecology of Sulfate Reducing Bacteria," *Producers Monthly, 22* (7), 17–29 (1958).
14. Brierley, J. A. and C. L. Brierley, "Biological Methods to Remove Selected Inorganic Pollutants from Uranium Mine Wastewater," in *Biogeochemistry of Ancient and Modern Environments,* P. A. Trudinger, M. R. Water, and B. J. Ralph, eds., Springer-Verlag, Berlin (1980).
15. Cork, D. J. and M. A. Cusanovich, "Sulfate Decomposition: A Microbial Process," in *Metallurgical Applications of Bacterial Leaching and Related Microbial Phenomena,* L. E. Murr, A. E. Torma, and J. A. Brierley, eds., Academic Press (1978).
16. Ebner, H. G., "Metal Recovery and Environmental Protection by Bacterial Leaching of Inorganic Waste Materials," in *Metallurgical Applications of Bacterial Leaching and Related Microbiological Phenomena,* L. E. Murr, A. E. Torma, and J. R. Brierley, eds., Academic Press (1978).
17. Carta, M., M. Ghiani, and G. Rossi, "Biochemical Beneficiation of Mining Industry Effluents," in *Biogeochemistry of Ancient and Modern Environments,* Springer-Verlag, Berlin (1980).

18. Solozhenkin, P. M. and L. Lyubavina, "The Bacterial Leaching of Antimony- and Bismuth-Bearing Ores and the Utilization of Sewage Waters," in *Biogeochemistry of Ancient Modern Environments,* Springer-Verlag, Berlin (1980).

19. Jeris, J. S. and R. W. Owens, "Pilot-Scale, High-Rate Biological Denitrification," *J. Water Poll. Control Fed., 47* (8), 2043–2057 (1975).

20. Cross, W. H., E. S. K. Chian, I. G. Rohland, S. Harper, S. Kharpar, S. S. Cheng, and F. Lu, "Anaerobic Biological Treatment of Coal Gasifier Effluent," *Biotechnology and Bioengineering, 12,* 349–363 (1982).

21. Lowhorn, R. W., R. B. Bustamante, and W. P. Bonner, "Carbon Removal and Nitrification in a Rotating Biological Contractor under Different Steady-State Conditions," Second Symposium on Biotechnology, in *Energy Production and Conservation,* John Wiley & Sons (1980).

22. Genung, R. K., C. W. Hancher, A. L. Rivera, and M. T. Harris, "Energy Conservation and Methane Production in Municipal Wastewater Treatment using Fixed-Film Anaerobic Bioreactors," *Biotechnology and Bioengineering Symposium, 12,* 365–380 (1982).

23. Genung, R. K., C. W. Hancher, M. T. Harris, and A. L. Rivera, "Pilot Scale Development of Fixed-Film Anaerobic Bioreactors for Municipal Wastewater Treatment," *AICHE Summer Natl. Meeting,* Cleveland, OH (1982).

24. Genung, R. H., M. T. Harris, A. L. Rivera, and T. L. Donaldson, "Operation of an Upflow Fixed-Bed Anaerobic Digester for Waste Stabilization and Fuel Gas Production at Near-Commercial Scale," *Energy from Biomass and Wastes VII,* Florida (1983).

25. Klibanov, A. M., T. Tu, and K. P. Scott, "Peroxidase-Catalyzed Removal of Phenols from Coal Conversion Waste Waters," *Science, 221,* 259–261 (1983).

26. Chakrabarty, A. M., "Genetic Mechanisms in Metal-Microbe Interactions," in *Applications of Bacterial Leaching and Related Microbiological Phenomena,* L. E. Murr, A. E. Torma, and J. A. Brierley, eds., Academic Press (1978).

10

Microbial Leaching of Metals

INTRODUCTION

The technology of microbial recovery of metals from ores dates back as early as 1000 B.C. The Romans extracted iron and copper sulfates from areas where natural sulfide leaching was taking place. The earliest records for large scale recovery of leached copper are from the Rio Tinto mines in Spain in the seventeenth and eighteenth centuries.

As with other biotechnologies (e.g., fermentation to produce food and beverages), the biological nature of the process of leaching was unknown to practitioners for many years. With the recognition of the role of microorganisms in leaching, considerable research and development has focused on the mechanisms of microbial leaching. This research extends from basic taxonomy (identifying the organisms involved) to laboratory tests and pilot scale investigations.

Biology of Microbial Leaching

The most important organisms involved in the leaching of metals are bacteria of the genus *Thiobacillus*, and in particular the species *Thiobacillus ferrooxidans*. These bacteria possess a combination of characteristics which allow them to function as catalysts in a series of reactions which lead to the release of metals from ore. The microorganisms obtain a large portion of their energy from the oxidation of inorganic substances. These oxidation reactions include the oxidation of sulfide minerals to soluble metal sulfates, and ferrous iron to the ferric form. A generalized reaction for the biological oxidation of mineral sulfide can be expressed as follows:

163

$$MS + 2O_2 \xrightarrow{\text{microorganism}} MSO_4$$

where M is a bivalent metal.

The *Thiobacilli* are acidophilic and thermophilic, tending to live in environments with a concentration of sulfuric acid and thriving in temperatures of between $20°$ and $35°C$. Another essential characteristic is the tolerance of the *Thiobacilli* to heavy metals at concentrations which are toxic to other microorganisms.

Since the discovery of the association between *T. ferrooxidans* and the dissolution of metals from ores, other species (e.g., *T. thiooxidans*) have been identified as important. Recent research has indicated the importance of mixed cultures in extracting certain ores which neither species alone can degrade.

Although it is clear that oxidation is the fundamental reaction in bacterial leaching, the exact nature of the process remains the subject of considerable research. One question is the relative importance of direct versus indirect oxidation. The direct process involves enzymatic attack on oxidizable components of the ore. By contrast, with indirect leaching the bacteria accelerate a natural process in which soluble ferrous iron is oxidized to ferric iron which, in turn, acts as an oxidizing agent for other metals. Ferrous iron is generated once again and the cycle is repeated.

Methods of Mining and Processing

There are four principal methods of leaching: dump, heap, *in situ*, and vat.

Dump leaching is used to extract metals from low-grade sulfide and oxide ores and run-off-the-mine waste materials. These materials are deposited in a valley with an impermeable base. Leach solutions are introduced at the top of the dump by spraying, flooding or injecting. The fluid percolates to the bottom where it is collected for subsequent metal recovery.

Heap leaching is similar to dump leaching, although smaller in scale, and is used primarily for crushed oxide ores with a higher metal concentration. As with dump leaching, water or an acidic solution is applied to the top of the heap and the solution that seeps to the bottom is recovered.

In situ leaching involves the pumping of leach solutions into abandoned mines, worked-out regions of mines or other below-ground cavities. The method of introducing the leach solution is dependent on the depth of the deposit in relation to the water table. *In situ* mining has the advantage, compared with dump and heap leaching, of reduced surface disturbance in terms of waste disposal and acid drainage. There is, however, an increased potential of groundwater contamination.

Vat leaching involves any process in which the bacterial leaching reactions occur in a confined tank. By controlling reaction conditions, leaching rates can be increased by several orders of magnitude over heap, dump, and *in situ* methods.

Metals can be recovered from leach solutions by a number of processes. Precipitation by iron cementation is the most commonly used commercial process. Alternatives include ion-exchange and solvent recovery. Electrolytic deposition (electrowinning) is used for solutions which contain higher concentrations of metals (e.g., those generated during vat leaching).

CURRENT INDUSTRIAL APPLICATIONS

Microbial leaching technologies are used commercially for two major applications: recovery of copper and uranium. As indicated earlier, microbial processes for copper recovery date back to 1000 B.C. and large-scale operations were established at the Rio Tinto mines in Spain as early as the 18th century. With the advent of nuclear technology, microbial leaching has also been applied to the recovery of uranium.

Copper Mining

Copper obtained through microbial leaching accounts for an estimated 10–15% of total U.S. copper production. Since the introduction of leaching technology in this country in 1914, dump, heap, and *in situ* processes have increased in size and number, principally in the Southwest. It was not until the early 1960s, however, that copper leaching processes were optimized. Prior to 1960, leaching processes consisted largely of precipitation of copper from acidified mine water or water which had passed through dumps. These operations were not subject to extensive design in terms of factors such as solution flow, chemical and biochemical kinetics, and aeration.

A number of factors led to an increased commercial interest in leaching technology over the past two decades. Trends in the minerals industry favoring leaching include the following:

• depletion of high-grade mineral resources
• tendency for mining to be extended deeper underground

- increasing volumes of low-grade waste accumulating in areas surrounding open-pit copper mines (estimated at nearly one million tons per day by 1980).

In addition, two general trends, rising energy costs and increasing concern over environmental pollution, are of particular importance to the copper industry. Hence, biological processes which use less energy (particularly fossil fuels) and result in less pollution are inherently attractive. Recent progress in genetic engineering technology has added another incentive for the use of microbial leaching.

The principal commercial methods of leaching are dump, heap and *in situ*. Acidic leach solutions are introduced at the top surface of an ore body and allowed to flow by gravity to a collection reservoir. The naturally occurring microorganisms in the ore body catalyze the oxidation reactions which release the minerals to the solution. The copper is then removed from solution by one of two processes:

- precipitation: a cementation reaction in which ferrous iron from scrap iron replaces the copper in solution;
- solvent extraction: in which an organic solvent is used to remove the copper from solution.

In both cases, the copper-free portion of the stream is replenished with acid or water, as appropriate, to adjust the pH and is recycled to the ore body. The copper-containing stream is then refined by electrowinning, smelting or other processes.

Uranium Mining

Microbial leaching of uranium is similar in many respects to leaching of copper. Both processes involve the recovery of metals from low-grade ores and/or abandoned mine workings, many of the same organisms are involved, the biochemical reactions are similar and the engineering design of leaching operations is fundamentally the same.

The conventional process for uranium recovery involves acid or carbonate leaching of finely ground ore followed by a solid-liquid separation step. The acidic waters contained significant quantities of uranium and also supported populations of the bacterium *Thiobacillus ferrooxidans*. Microbially assisted leaching was recognized in the early 1960s as a potentially beneficial process, rather than simply a pollution problem, and high pressure hosing of mine slopes was commenced in 1963 in Canada. Since that time, the growth of microbial uranium leaching has been limited by a number of factors and the conventional methods still predominate.

The role of bacteria in the extraction of uranium from its ore appears to be an indirect one: generating an oxidant which then attacks the mineral and creating the acid solution which removes it in solution. Direct enzymatic attack is not involved in uranium leaching reactions.

The oxidation-reduction reactions in uranium leaching are similar to those for copper leaching. *T. ferrooxidans* oxidizes ferrous iron and pyrite to produce the oxidant, ferric iron and sulfuric acid. Ferric iron attacks minerals containing guadrivalent uranium (U^{4+})and oxidizes this to hexavalent uranium (U^{6+}) which is soluble in the sulfuric acid.

Other Metals

The solubilization of valuable metal from ores by bacteria means has been investigated in the laboratory for many metals. Some results are summarized in Table 10-1 for important metals.

CONCLUSIONS

This chapter has demonstrated the interest in using microorganisms in extractive metallurgy and the commercial success achieved in copper and uranium extraction.

TABLE 10-1. Results from Microbial Leaching Experiments.

Metal Recovery	Organism	Temperature	pH	Percent
Tin	T. ferrooxidans	30–40 °C	2.5	97.3% in 15 days
Potassium	Scopulariopsis brevicaule			some solubilization
Bismuth	T. ferrooxidans T. Thiooxidans	37 °C		90% in 4 days
Aluminum	Silicate bacteria Fungi	32 °C	7.0	21–33% in 30 days
Molybdenum	Chemoautotrophic org. from thermal spring	60 °C		13.3% in 30 days
Zinc	T. ferrooxidans	30 °C	2.5	>95% in 5 days
Cadmium	T. ferrooxidans	35 °C	2.3	>95%
Nickel	T. ferrooxidans Beijerinckia lactinogenes			>40%
	Thermophilic bacteria	50 °C		95% in 35 days
Vanadium	T. ferrooxidans		1.0	30%
Arsenic	T. ferrooxidans			97% in 6 days
Antimony	Sulfite reducing bacteria	37.5 °C		90%
Manganese	Many organisms			

Extensive research in the microbiology of leaching of ores of diverse quality and origin is being conducted by universities, government agencies and commercial firms. This research indicates a growing interest in expanding the domain of microbial leaching technology.

Dollars are the great equalizers and the great common denominators. The future of commercial microbial leaching will depend on comprehensive analyses of the comparative economics (both external and internalized costs) of microbial leaching and traditional hydrometallurgies.

The new science of biotechnology (especially recombinant DNA technology) will be called upon to play a major role in expanding the range of applications of microbial leaching. Already, a number of plasmids from *Thiobacillus* have been mapped and spliced into *Eschericha coli* and in other host organisms. An extensive program of characterization, mapping and sequencing of appropriate genes would provide the necessary data base for a systematic use of existing material and for the design of organisms with enhanced or new capabilities.

Based on this survey, a number of simple forecasts can be made for the immediate future in North America:

• As the quality of available ore decreases and as the cost of mineral extraction increases, microbial leaching systems will become more important.
• An increasing number of microbial leaching systems will move from the laboratory to pilot tests and, eventually, full scale operations.
• Recombinant DNA will play a more important role in designing the most effective microbial extraction systems.
• The basic knowledge gained in microbial leaching studies will be applied to using microorganisms and enzymes for metal solubilization, precipitation, valence changes (through oxydo reduction mechanisms), and binding to organic materials.
• A combination of chemical and biological leaching processes and metal recovery will be more effective than each working alone. Hybrid systems will take advantage of the best features of the two technologies.
• New microbial systems from hostile environments (hot springs, undersea vents, acid mine drainage pools, soils) will be tested in the laboratory on a variety of ores and waste.
• Biological systems which function at higher temperature will be exploited.
• Mixed groups of biological organisms working in symbiosis will be emphasized.

The above predictions assume an economy in which the demand for metals is sufficient to allow research and development by the mining and primary metals industries. The most recent recession has had the effect of limiting such R&D investment.

The most important hurdle for any new industrial process to penetrate the marketplace is the demonstration of technical and economic feasibility. Microbial leaching technology draws from several well partitioned disciplines: biology, geology, and engineering. Because of the need to speak several "languages" simultaneously, progress has been slow. The need is apparent for a training program marrying the required disciplines.

The survey indicates that in spite of considerable research, the process of microbial leaching is still not well understood in terms of the underlying physical, chemical and biological mechanisms. A return to fundamentals would provide a stronger base upon which a large scale commercial edifice can be built.

11

Separation, Concentration, Purification and Products Recovery Techniques in Biotechnology

INTRODUCTION

S*eparation processes are* defined as those unit operations which trans-form a mixture of components into two or more product streams which differ from one another in composition. Product recovery is defined as the quantitative extraction of a specific chemical entity from a mixture. Concentration is the removal of water from an aqueous solution or some other solvent in order to obtain a more concentrated product. Purification is the improvement in purity of a product.

Distillation is the most widely used separation, concentration, and purification technique; with the aid of energy input in the form of heat, two phases are created: a vapor phase and a liquid phase. The suitability of distillation as a separation, purification, and concentration method is strongly dependent on favorable vapor-liquid equilibrium, feed composition, number of components to be separated, product purity, the absolute pressure, heat sensitivity, and corrosivity. The alternative separation processes of industrial importance are the following:

Membrane Methods
   Reverse Osmosis
   Ultrafiltration
   Microfiltration
   Liquid Membranes
   Electrodialysis
   Gas Separation

Mechanical Methods
   Ultracentrifugation
   Filtration

Liquid-Gas-Solid Extraction Methods
  Adsorption
  Absorption
  Chromatography
  Solvent Extraction
  Supercritical fluid extraction

Heat Treatments
  Distillation
  Evaporation
  Drying Systems
  Freeze Crystallization

Electric/Magnetic Methods
  Electrophoresis
  Electromagnetic Separation
  Electrofiltration
  Electro Coagulation
  Electrostatic Separation
  Electro Magnetic Energy Dryers

Separation, as the generic term, means selection based on differential properties between the substance of interest and other present and interfering substances. Selection can be made on the basis of size, weight, solubility, electrostatic or magnetic properties, ability to bind to ligand, etc. A force is applied to achieve separation. For instance, gravity is the force involved in sedimentation, centrifugal forces control separation by centrifugation, an electric field assures partition by electrophoresis, a magnetic field explains high gradient magnetic separation, reverse osmosis, ultrafiguration and microfiltration are all pressure driven processes. Sometimes more than one force is involved: electrodialysis is basically an electricity augmented pressure driven process and electric focusing combines a pH gradient and an electric field. Any attempt to classify processes in mutually exclusive and exhaustive categories is doomed to fail. Much overlap and combinations exist between the methods, techniques and processes described below.

Biotechnology involves unique unit operations such as fermentation, special material such as live cells and unusual and specialized products, such as enzymes. For the most part, downward processing in biotechnology is quite similar to established technologies in use in the chemical, pharmaceutical, petroleum and food industry. While many unique biotechnology separation and recovery methods have been tested only at the laboratory level; other processes are well demonstrated at the pilot plant and full scale level. The first group offers a limited range of solutions; the second group a wide range of proven concepts and devices.

Product separation and purification pose special problems in biotechnology. Many bioproducts are fragile. Products are usually dissolved in large quantities of water or held in cells. In some cases, the microbial cells are themselves the desired product. Multiple products of many bioreactions must be separated without destruction, molecular rearrangement, loss of activity, or interference.

Product separation costs vary according to the application, but are usually the main cost factor in any industrial process. To address these problems and reduce the contribution of downstream processing to total cost, methods are needed that have some or all of the following characteristics:

* high product recovery;
* reliability and insensitivity to variations in stream quality;
* ability to process in pace with reactor production (i.e., minimal storage or holdup);
* little or no modification of the activity of the compound;
* low cost and energy requirements; and
* capability for recycling of medium or biological catalyst.

To meet these requirements on a full commercial scale for a range of applications, new techniques are under development and some existing techniques (e.g., distillation) are being modified for increased efficiency and suitability to biological process streams.

One of the difficulties associated with a new emerging technology is a tendency to reinvent well established technologies rather than adapt well proven methods from neighboring fields. The converse is equally true: a custom made technology, for a specific situation, can be stretched only so much to fit a novel application. One solution is to return to first principles (physics and chemistry) in attempting to develop purification, separation and concentration solutions applicable to biotechnology.

The field of separation techniques is vast and expanding with each new application attempted and each new problem solved. It is not possible to be comprehensive. The review will emphasize those techniques which are likely to be applied to a wide variety of problems in the future. A touristic view of the wealth of methods in use is presented. The emphasis is on membrane methods with the greatest potential for application to difficult biotechnology separation problems.

MEMBRANE METHODS

Separation methods based on membrane technology are probably the most applicable to biotechnology. Their selectivity, their gentle treatment of the material, and the ability of the membranes to be manufactured and formed in a variety of shapes give them great flexibility. Six processes of broad interest to the biotechnologist are described:

Process	Material Selected	Driving Force	Material Retained
Reverse Osmosis	Water	Pressure	Essentially all suspended & dissolved species
Ultrafiltration	Water & salts	Pressure	Organic material above a MW cutoff point
Microfiltration	Water & dissolved species	Pressure	All material above a size cutoff point
Electrodialysis	Ions	Pressure & electric current	All nonionic species
Liquid-Liquid Membranes	Chemical	Solubility Active transport	Water Other chemical species
Gas Separation	Specific gases	Pressure	Other gases & vapor

Reverse Osmosis

Reverse osmosis (RO) is a pressure-driven process in which salt, low molecular weight organic molecules, and ionic species 1×100^{-2} um in diameter and less than 300 molecular weight are retained [1]. Since ionic species are retained by the membrane, reverse osmosis processes are operated at relatively high pressures (100 to 2000 psi, 0.69 to 13.8 MPa) to overcome osmotic pressure of the retentate and thus drive the permeate fluid through the membrane. The driving force responsible for the fluid flow is osmotic pressure. The pressure magnitude is dependent upon membrane characteristics, water temperature and salt solution concentration. By applying pressure to the saline water, the flow through the membrane can be reversed. Whenever the applied pressure on the salt solution is greater than the osmotic pressure, fresh water diffuses through the membrane and pure solvent is extracted from the mixed solution.

RO is fundamentally a method for separating dissolved solids from water molecules in aqueous solutions as a result of the characteristic membranes composed of special polymers which allow water molecules to pass through while holding back most other types of molecules. In an actual reverse osmosis system, operating in a continuous flow process, feedwater to be treated is circulated through an input passage of the cell, separated from the output product water passageway by the membrane. The input stream is divided into two fractions—a purified portion called the product water or permeate, and a smaller portion called the concentrate, containing most of the chemical species in the feedstream. At the far end of the feedwater passage, the concentration (dewatered) reject stream exits from the cell. After permeating the membrane, the product (freshwater) flow is collected. The percentage of product water obtained from the feedstream is termed the recovery, and is typically around 75%.

This process requires a dense membrane, since for all intents, the pores are non-existent. However, a membrane suitably dense for the rejection of ionic species would, if it were thick, greatly retard the flux of the permeate. Therefore, reverse osmosis membranes used to have a very thin dense skin covering a very porous structure which permits passage of the permeate while providing needed structural support [2].

Loeb-Sourirajan thin-skinned anisotropic membranes are the major membranes in reverse osmosis applications. After the reverse osmosis membrane has been formed, it is annealed in hot water to tighten the membrane by increasing its density. This process causes an increase in salt rejection and a decrease in water flux with an increase in annealing temperature. The membranes are generally cast as flat-sheet stock or as hollow fibers. Reverse osmosis hollow fibers are cast with the thin, dense skin on the outside of the fiber so that the permeate passes into the lumen of the tube. This fact, coupled with the smaller cross-sectional area of reverse osmosis membranes compared to ultrafiltration membranes, makes them better able to withstand the compressional forces of the higher pressure of reverse osmosis [3].

Composite membranes are very thin but dense membranes deposited over a porous supporting substrate. These membranes are produced by first making a fine microporous membrane substrate by dissolving a non-water-soluble polymer in an organic solvent and then casting this solution in air or in water. A high degree of control is exacted during manufacture over both pore size and membrane ultrastructure. A thin film of material, such as cellulose triacetate or polyethylene imine, is applied to the supporting membrane surface. For successful operation, the supporting membrane pore diameter must be less than the film thickness (0.05 to 0.1 um) to assure that the entire membrane is film coated, and has a sufficiently high porosity to maintain the required water flux. The advantages of composite membranes include their ability to utilize thin films made of polymers that cannot be fabricated into Loeb-Sourirajan membranes, and a high degree of control over film thickness and its reproducibility. The membrane substrate can be fabricated of materials that exhibit resistance to membrane compaction under the pressures of reverse osmosis.

Dynamically formed membranes are fabricated by coating a porous carbon, ceramic, or metallic tube with coloidal zirconium oxide, poly-acrylic acid, or with the suspended material in the effluent stream itself. These membranes tend to have higher flux and lower rejection than conventional reverse osmosis membranes and they can operate at high temperatures (85 °C) [4].

There are three types of commercially available membranes: cellulose acetate, aromatic polyamide, and composite membranes variously fabricated. The performance of cellulose-acetate membrane is related to the annealing temperature, with lower flux and higher rejection rates at higher temperatures. Such membranes are prone to hydrolysis at extreme pH, subject to compaction at operating pressures, and sensitive to free chlorine above 1.0 ppm. Cellulose acetate membranes are further biodegradable and susceptible to hydrolyzation by acids and alkalis. Cellulose acetate membranes generally have a useful life of two to three years. Aromatic polyamide membranes are prone to compaction. The fibers are more resistant to hydrolysis than cellulose acetate membranes but they are more sensitive to free chlorine. Composite membranes of poly (ether/amide) generally exhibit a higher water flux and salt rejection than cellulose acetate. They are very sensitive to free chlorine [2].

The vast majority of industrial applications use either spiral-wound modules fabricated from sheet stock or hollow fibers. Hollow fibers are particularly prone to fouling and, once fouled, they are hard to clean. Thus, applications which employ these fibers require a great deal of pretreatment to remove all suspended and colloidal material in the feed stream. Spiral-wound modules, due to their relative resistance to fouling, have a broader range of applications. A major advantage of the hollow fiber modules, however, is the fact that a hollow-fine-fiber module can pack 5,000 square feet (465 square meters) of surface area in a one cubic foot (0.028 cubic meter) volume, while a spiral wound module can only contain 300 square feet (27.9 square meters) in the same volume. A third type is the tubular system. It is essentially a stainless steel tube with the membrane coated or inserted inside the tube. The sintered stainless steel tubes with dynamically formed membranes are formed from powdered metals and have micropores (0.5 um). They are located in bundles inside 8–10 in. pipes. Their special interest is their ability to operate at high pressure (1,200 psi) without membrane compaction and at high temperature (100 °C). Tube systems are not susceptible to fouling but are several times more costly than spiral-wound membranes [5].

Major problems inherent in most applications of reverse osmosis are associated with the presence of particulate and colloidal matter in feedwater; precipitation of soluble salts; and physical and chemical makeup of the feedwater. In order to mitigate against concentration polarization, a high rate of fluid cross-flow is maintained to reduce the effective thickness of the boundary layer. However, in reverse osmosis, the ultimate objective is to remove as much pure water from the feed stream as possible which in turn, due to significant volume reduction, serves to reduce the rate of flow of the feed stream over the membrane surface. This additional problem is often mitigated by a "tapered" arrangement of membrane modules. Fouling of membranes, either by precipitated solutes in the boundary layer, micro-organisms, or particulates in the feed stream, tends to reduce membrane flux and to eventually render the membranes irreparably inoperative [2].

The advantages of reverse osmosis membranes are primarily related to comparative economics by comparison with single purpose multistage distillation (although this advantage evaporates when compared to both triple-effect evaporation and vapor recovery) and to the relatively high rates of flux and ion rejection found in most reverse osmosis membranes in commercial use. Two of the major operating costs of reverse osmosis plants are electrical power and membrane replacement. The high operating pressures of reverse osmosis (100 to 2,000 psi, 0.69 to 13.8 MPa) require relatively large amounts of electrical energy. With the rapidly escalating costs of energy in recent years, the energy component of reverse osmosis operating costs has taken on an increasingly important role. Reverse osmosis membranes must be replaced relatively frequently due to loss of water flux over time as a result of compaction; fouling of membranes or modules to the extent that chemical or physical cleaning can no longer restore sufficient levels of water flux; and actual degradation of the membrane due to hydrolysis, extremes of pH, or the action of free chlorine [2].

Reverse osmosis and ultrafiltration are similar in that they are both pressure-driven processes and they both separate a feed stream into a product stream and a reject stream. The differences between these two processes are important and include the following [2].

- The size of the molecules retained by the membrane differs between the two processes with the actual boundary depending upon the specific membrane. Generally, reverse osmosis membranes have a molecular weight cutoff of less than 300 while ultrafiltration membranes have a 300 to 300,000 molecular weight cutoff.
- Reverse osmosis is generally used to separate ionic species from a solution. This results in formation of an often considerable osmotic gradient across the membrane due to the differential ionic concentra-

tions of the fluids on each side of the membrane. Osmotic pressure is a negligible consideration in most applications of ultrafiltration systems.

• Operating pressures are considerably higher in reverse osmosis than they are in ultrafiltration systems. Therefore, in reverse osmosis the thin membrane skin is on the outside of the fiber and pressure is applied on the outside so that the fiber is subject to compression rather than tension.

• In reverse osmosis, the membrane serves primarily as a diffusive transport barrier, and as such, the actual chemistry of the membrane plays a key role in determining the rejection of various molecules. Although molecular screening may play a possible role in reverse osmosis membrane retention, it is the prime mechanism in ultrafiltration processes [6].

Reverse osmosis should find many applications in biotechnology. For instance, hollow fiber systems, when applied to fermentation broths, have achieved high concentration factors (greater than 90% solids by volume) at rapid filtration rates (up to 1 liter/min/ft² of membrane area). This method provides an inexpensive technique for cell harvesting.

Ultrafiltration

In ultrafiltration (UF), an emulsion is introduced into and pumped through a membrane. Water and some dissolved low molecular weight materials pass through the membrane under the applied hydrostatic pressure. Emulsified droplets and suspended particles are retained, concentrated and removed continuously as a fluid concentrate. In contrast to ordinary filtration, there is no build-up of retained materials on the membrane filter.

The pore structure of the membrane acts as a filter, passing small solutes such as salts, while retaining larger emulsified and suspended material. The pores of ultrafiltration membranes are much smaller than the particles rejected, and particles cannot enter the membrane structure. As a result, the pores cannot become plugged. Pore structure and size (less than 0.005 microns) of ultrafiltration membranes are quite different from those of ordinary filters in which pore plugging results in drastically reduced filtration rates and requires frequent backflushing or some other regeneration step.

Ultrafiltration utilizes membranes with small pore sizes ranging from 0.015 to 8 microns in order to collect small particles, to separate small particles according to sizes or to obtain particle-free solutions. UF membranes are characterized by smallness and uniformity of pore size, difficult to achieve with cellulosic filters. They are further characterized by thinness, strength, flexibility, low absorption and adsorption and a flat surface texture. These properties are useful for a variety of analytical and separation procedures.

Particles larger than the actual pore size of the membrane are captured by filtration on the surface. Total surface retention makes it possible to determine, quantitatively by weight or by chemical analysis, the amount and type of particles in either liquids or gases. Since there are no tortuous paths in the membrane to entrap particles smaller than the pore size, particles can be separated into various size ranges by serial filtration through membranes with successively smaller pore sizes.

Fluids and gases may be cleaned by passing them through a membrane filter with a pore size small enough to prevent passage of specific contaminants. This capability is especially useful in a variety of process industries which require cleaning or sterilization of fluids and gases. The retention efficiency of membranes is dependent on particle size and concentration; membrane pore size, length, and porosity; and overall flow rate.

In contrast to reverse osmosis, where cellulose acetate membranes occupy a predominant position; a variety of synthetic polymers have been employed for ultrafiltration membranes. Many of these membranes can be handled dry, have superior organic solvent resistance and are less sensitive to temperature and pH than cellulose acetate. Polycarbonate resins, substituted olefins and polyelectrolyte complexes have been employed among other polymers to form ultrafiltration membranes [2].

Molecular weight cutoff is used as a measure of rejection; shape, size and flexibility are also important parameters. For a given molecular weight, more rigid molecules are better rejected than flexible ones. Ionic strength and pH often help determine the shape and rigidity of large molecules. Maximum operating temperatures for membranes with 5,000–10,000 mol wt. cutoffs are about 65 °C. For a 50,000–80,000 mol wt. cutoff, maximum operating temperatures are in the 50 °C range.

Ultrafiltration (UF), electrodialysis (ED) and reverse osmosis (RO) can be used advantageously at several points in an alcohol from biomass plant. The dilute feedstock can be concentrated by UF or RO prior to fermentation. UF can be applied to the beer to produce distillers dried grain and a clear permeate for distillation. Treatment of the UF permeate by ED can remove excess salts. This deionized liquid can be treated by RO to produce pure water for recycling. UF can be used to allow higher yeast cell in the fermenter and remove alcohol from the fermenter, hence accelerating the alcohol production [7]. The introduction of proteases (papain, fungal proteinase) unto ultrafiltration membranes serves as a self-cleaning method and increase permeate flux [8].

Ultrafiltration processes have a number of advantages that they share to some degree with microfiltration processes [2].

- Ultrafiltration is an athermal process and, if necessary, can operate at relatively low temperature to insure preservation of heat-sensitive materials.
- No phase change, such as in freezing or evaporation, is required for separation or concentration of materials by ultrafiltration. This process is not only gentle on the materials to be separated or concentrated, but in most cases it also saves the energy that would otherwise be required to accomplish the phase change.
- Relatively low hydrostatic pressures are used in ultrafiltration processes, compared to reverse osmosis. High pressure can lead to membrane compaction or even rupture. These lower pressures are relatively gentle and use less energy.
- No chemical reagents or catalysts are required to operate ultrafiltration processes. Although in many instances detergents, chlorine, sodium hydroxide, and other chemical agents are used to clean fouled membranes. It is possible to backflush the membrane with permeate.
- Ultrafiltration processes permit the simultaneous concentration and purification of process and/or product streams, reducing the complexity of process design and equipment and, in many cases, reducing energy requirements.
- Ultrafiltration processes maintain a constant pH in the concentrate stream and (unlike reverse osmosis) also maintain a constant ionic strength.
- Economics are generally favorable for ultrafiltration systems. Microfiltration systems usually have more surface area and longer membrane life than ultrafiltration systems, but this longer life is a result of lower flux of permeate through the membrane. The two prime economic considerations are membrane replacement costs and utility costs. Although reverse osmosis modules are among the cheapest available, the rising world energy costs are such that the cost of utilities is rapidly becoming a key factor in process consideration.
- Ultrafiltration membranes are particularly well suited to the concentration of enzyme products, since the relatively low temperatures and the relatively gentle shear forces in thin-channel systems mitigate the tendency of enzymes to become inactivated. Other applications for ultrafiltration include concentration of viruses and separation of biochemicals produced by enzymatic processes in enzyme reactors where enzymes are actually adsorbed on the surface of the membrane. In many pharmaceutical applications, it is important to

sterilize the membrane. Depending upon the membrane composition, a variety of methods may be employed including the use of formaldehyde, ethanol, ethylene oxide, and autoclaving.

Microfiltration

Microfiltration (MF) is a pressure-driven process allowing the retention of particulates, organisms, colloids and viruses generally in the 0.02 to 10 um size range or greater than 300,000 molecular weight [1]. There are two basic types of microfiltration membranes fundamentally different in their manufacture and structure; the tortuous-pore membrane and the capillary-pore membrane. Their differences are reflected in the different applications in which these membranes are used.

Tortuous-pore membranes consist of a polymer matrix surrounding numerous interconnected vacuoles that results in convoluted pathways through the membrane matrix material. The most common technique for manufacture of tortuous-pore microfiltration membranes involves a phase-inversion casting process in which the relative amounts of polymer, solvent and water, as well as drying rates, are all controlled to determine the number and size of the vacuoles in the polymer matrix. A consequence of this type of casting is the characteristics of the channels arising from interconnected vacuoles. The channels are not uniform in width, and there are constrictions along the channels path. The diameter of the channels at these constrictions limits the size of the particle or material which can pass through the membrane. These channels are not linear but rather follow convoluted and interconnected pathways, hence the name "tortuous pore" [2].

Capillary-pore membranes are produced by a technique that produces straight-channel cylindrical pores with uniform diameter. These membranes are manufactured in a two-stage process. In the first stage, a film of polycarbonate, polyester, or polypropylene is subjected to bombardment by energetic nuclei which leave a thin trail of radiation-damaged material throughout the film. In the second stage, the film is subjected to an etching process that selectively dissolves that portion of the film that has been damaged. The etching process leaves cylindrical, straight pores through the membrane material [9]. This process insures a high degree of control over the characteristics of the membrane. The number of pores per unit area is a function of the number of high energy nuclei which bombarded the film. The etching process is independent of the radiation exposure and, by varying the temperature, concentration, and residence time in the etch bath, the pore size can be controlled.

Both types of membranes exhibit total retention of all particles larger than the specified pore size and are thus amenable to use for sterilization or other applications that would require complete particles or organisms removal. Both types of membranes can be autoclaved at least once. The capillary-pore membranes made of polycarbonate can be autoclaved repeatedly [2].

Given a membrane with a particular pore size for filtration of a sample containing variable-sized particles, different capture mechanisms apply to the different particle sizes [9,10]. Very small particles, having relatively high diffusion coefficients, are captured on the membrane surface or on the internal pore surface by adsorption following diffusion to the membrane surface. For relatively large particles, impaction on the pore lip is the dominant mechanism. Impaction on the pore lip or inner surface of the pore near the lip results when the mass of the particle is sufficiently large to carry it across the fluid viscous-flow stream lines of material through the pore.

The differences between capillary-pore membranes and tortuous-pore membranes may be important in specific applications [2]:

- tortuous-pore membranes have a porosity of about 80% while capillary-pore membranes generally have a porosity of only 10%;
- the capillary-pore membranes are only about one-twelfth the thickness of the tortuous pore membranes; and
- the capillary-pore membranes are highly flexible and thus can be pleated into cartridges.

The high porosity of tortuous pore membranes is of particular utility in:

- cases where organisms must be cultured and collected on the membrane surface, particularly when nutrients are to be transmitted through the pores from below the membrane; and
- in membrane electrophoresis when molecules must migrate across the membrane diameter in an electric field.

The low porosity and uniformly flat surface of the capillary pore membranes are particularly advantageous in applications such as:

- microscopic analysis of material collected on the surface of the membrane (which would tend to be imbedded below the surface in tortuous-pore networks); and
- where staining is required to count organisms such as bacteria (since the polycarbonate film does not stain).

The thin and straight channels in capillary-pore membranes are important in several applications.

- Concentration and/or purification of biological agents, such as viruses, is more cost-effective with capillary-pore membranes because far less material is lost due to adsorption on the walls of the capillary tube than would adsorb into the tortuous channels.

- Capillary-pore membranes are particularly useful in cases where one wants to fractionate a sample containing particles of different sizes. The small particles have less surface area for adsorption in the capillary pores than they would in the tortuous pores where significant portion of the sample could be lost.

The most common applications of microfiltration membranes are dictated by their ability to retain all of the particles above a specified size and by their retention of particles greater than 300,000 molecular weight and in the 0.02 to 10 um size range. Thus, microfiltration membranes are used in applications where organisms and particulate material removal is of primary concern, such as sterilization and harvesting of cellular material in the pharmaceutical industry. Most of these specific applications are small-scale uses and laboratory applications, with the exceptions of brewery, wine, and soft drink sterilization.

Initially microfiltration got its start in microbiology with the development of microfiltration membranes that would retain bacterial organisms which were cultured and counted on the surface of the membrane. This application is in widespread use in laboratories. Industrial applications of microfiltration are largely extensions of its laboratory applications. Specific examples include:

- removal of particulates and other material causing turbidity in serum;
- removal of stroma and particulate material during the collection of hemoglobin;
- concentration of yeast and bacteria used in the biological production of enzymes and pharmaceuticals;
- fractionation of enzymes; and
- yeast removal from liquid sugar.

A promising use for microfiltration systems is in the cold sterilization of beer and wine. Yeasts and bacteria are removed from the product without the use of heat which could alter the taste of the beer or wine. Only one brewery in the United States is currently sterilizing draft beer by means of microfiltration [2].

Advantages and disadvantages depend upon the specific application and type of membrane. The most important considerations include the following [2].

- A relatively high initial cost of microfiltration systems which is offset by lower operating costs due to a reduced need to replace filter elements compared to ultrafiltration and reverse osmosis.

- Microfiltration membranes have a sharper molecular weight cutoff than other membrane types and can effectively retain all of a given particle size. These features permit applications requiring sample fractionation and/or sterilization.
- Capillary-pore membranes, because of their smooth surface and straight cylindrical pores, have a much lower capacity to retain particles than do tortuous-pore membranes. However, since capillary-pore membranes can be pleated and inserted into cartridges which provide a large surface area in a small space, this lack of capacity can be offset.

Liquid Membranes

Most of the natural and artificial membranes that are commercially used are solids made up of polymeric materials. Separation technologies based on these membranes are sometimes inefficient for two reasons: diffusion coefficients in solid polymeric materials tend to be low and the membranes are not always highly selective.

Liquid membranes are of two types: support-type and emulsion-type. The liquid membrane with support utilizes a microporous membrane where pores are filled with liquid. The liquid membrane without support, also known as a liquid-surfactant membrane (emulsion type), can be operational when the membrane forms tiny droplets suspended in a liquid phase. Li developed the separation technique using liquid surfactant membrane in emulsified solutions [11]. An aqueous solution of surfactant is placed at the bottom of a separation column. On top of the surfactant solution, an organic solvent occupies a space through which tiny droplets rise. The feed solution is introduced at the bottom of the column. As the surfactant droplets containing the feed pass through the solvent phase, selective permeation takes place through the thin liquid membrane. As the droplets reach the top of the solvent phase, they are enriched with less permeating components and coalesce to form a product solution. Liquid membranes are capable of moving a particular solute from a region of high concentration into a region of low concentration. A liquid membrane can separate two miscible liquids and can control the mass transfer between these liquids [12].

Liquid membranes, in general, are formed by making an emulsion of two immiscible phases and then dispersing the emulsion in a third phase (the continuous phase). There are two major types of emulsion type liquid membrane systems. One is a water-immiscible emulsion dispersed in water and the other is an oil-immiscible emulsion dispersed in oil. These emulsions consist of an encapsulating phase composed of surfactants, various additives, and a base material. For example, the oil phase encapsulates microscopic droplets of an aqueous solution of appropriate reagents for removing and trapping the material that is extracted. The surfactants and additives are used to control the stability, permeability and selectivity of the membrane. In the liquid membrane process, the aqueous solutin is distributed as small droplets within larger drops of solvent. This gives the benefit of the thin solvent membrane in a form where a large interfacial area is more easily achieved. The process also provides a kind of extraction phenomenon in which the solute capacity of a dispersed solvent is increased by addition of islands of an irreversibly reactive material [13].

The three main types of diffusion that can occur through liquid membranes are simple passive diffusion down a gradient in concentration or thermodynamic activity, facilitated transport (in this process, a carrier agent capable of combining with the permeate to be transported is dissolved in the liquid membrane phase); and coupled transport processes. In this last case, the carrier agent couples the flow of two or more species. Because of this coupling, one of the species can be moved against its concentration gradient, provided the concentration gradient of the second coupled species is sufficiently large.

A facilitated transport or carrier transport mechanism can be used to enhance the mass transfer. This is achieved by incorporating a reagent in the encapsulated phase that can react with the permeating compound from the continuous aqueous phase; or a compound, such as a complexing agent, in the membrane phase to increase the solubility of the permeating compound in the membrane, thus increasing the permeation rate of this compound through the membrane.

Liquid membranes [14] like biomembranes, can be made highly fluid and, because of their low viscosity, exhibit low diffusivities. Both types of membranes can behave as "chemical pumps." Liquid membranes are attractive separation tools where speed and selectivity are paramount, but the cost more than distillation or fractional crystallization. Liquid membranes can be made extremely selective, thin, reusable, and inexpensive to operate.

Liquid membrane permeation can be used to separate hydrocarbon mixtures as well as aqueous solutions. The separation of the feed mixture can be achieved based on the difference of the permeation rates of the feed components. The individual permeation rates tend to vary with temperature, agitation speed, and film composition. In conventional separation methods, such as distillation, solvent extraction, and adsorption, the equilibrium distribution can be approached with reboil and reflux. In contrast, permeation is a separation based on relative rates of transfer of two components between two liquid phases separated by a membrane. During this separation, transfer of the components is in one direction only, i.e., from feed to solvent.

Biochemical and biomedical separations include the use of liquid membranes in preparing medicinals, oxygenation of blood, treatment of chronic uremia and emergency treatment of drug overdose. The membranes can also be used in the reverse mode: a useful drug or enzyme may be encapsulated in the internal phase of the liquid membrane for later slow or controlled release of the drug. Successful immobilization of enzymes by liquid for membrane encapsulation has been accomplished with phenolase, urease, amylase, lipase, lactase, and trypsin, among others. These encapsulated enzymes can be used to facilitate enzyme-induced chemical reactions, and in preparing chemicals and pharmaceutical preparations.

In addition to separation applications there are other important liquid membrane applications: immobilized liquid membrane electrodes, controlled release and multiple emulsion.

Immobilized liquid membrane electrodes use liquid ion-exchangers or other carriers (e.g., ionophores), typically immobilized in a plasticized polyvinyl chloride membrane or the pores of a microporous membrane. These electrodes are used as pH, ions or gas sensors and are expected to find great use in the detection and measurement of a variety of chemicals. The key is to identify highly specific reactions that convert the species to be analyzed into a species readily detected by an existing ion-selective electrode. The immobilized liquid in these cases contains an enzyme which is a highly specific catalyst for a chemical reaction.

Controlled release technology deals with the regulation of the rate at which biologically active substances are released to their environment. This technology allows the user to stretch out the time over which the concentration of the substance remains above an effective threshold level. Applications of immobilized liquid membranes are currently being developed in the pharmaceutical, agricultural, and chemical industries, as well as for insect and pest control.

In the U.K., multiple emulsion systems were preferred vehicles for the administration of certain vaccines during the 1960s. Up until that time, the simple water/oil emulsions had been used but these were difficult to inject through a hypodermic needle. The multiple emulsion system for the administration of pharmacological agents was patented about this time [15]. The drug in aqueous solution is contained in the internal phase and thereby is released slowly through the oil layer to give a sustained release system [16]. The multiple emulsion system has been shown to have far better delivery capabilities than simple water/oil emulsion systems.

Pervaporation is a technique incorporating the selective sorption of a liquid mixture, diffusion of molecules through the membrane, and desorption into a vapor phase on a downstream side of a membrane.

Permeselectivity and permeability of the membrane are involved. Concentration is the driving force. The method has been successfully applied to separating trace organics from a dilute environment [17].

Gas Separation

Gas separation by semipermeable membranes is also a pressure-drive process that depends upon differential permeability of certain membranes to different gases [18]. Membranes used for gas separation processes are basically similar to those used in reverse osmosis and they are configured into modules similar to those employed in other pressure-driven filtration processes. There are three major types of gas separation membranes commercially available at this time, each of which is typically used in a particular modular configuration [2].

* Thin-skinned anisotropic cellulose acetate membranes were shown to have high flux to gases with relatively high selectivity to different gas molecules. Commercial dry Loeb-Sourirajan membranes are fabricated into spiral-wound modules from flat membrane stock.
* A recently developed membrane for gas separation consists of a thin, cast, supporting film of silicone rubber coated with a highly permeable polymer film. These membranes are used in plate and frame modules for oxygen enrichment of air for medical applications.
* A hollow-fiber filter of polysulfone coated with a non-selective, highly permeable polymer film such as silicone rubber. The fibers are fabricated into tubular modules up to 20 feet (6.1 meters) in length and represent a significant advancement in gas separation technology because they possess both high flux and high gas molecule separation.

The most important operational considerations for membrane gas separation applications are the relative fluxes and separation efficiency. For efficient operation of a gas separation process it is desirable to have a high gas flux through the membrane as well as a high degree of separation of gas molecules. This has not been the case in practice with most gas separation membranes; separation has been inversely proportional to membrane permeability.

Membrane gas separation is just beginning to be commercialized, thus many apparent disadvantages are being, or soon will be, overcome. The problem of the inversely proportional relationship between gas flux and separation has recently been overcome with the development of hollow fine fibers for gas separations. Gas separation has an operating cost advantage in that in many applications the feed stream is already pressurized. The resulting permeate gas can be used without the necessity of recompression. The savings of energy cost inherent in the pressurized product can be a considerable advantage. Gas separation reverse osmosis membrane processes are the newest of the membrane separation processes, and they have only been of commercial importance for a few years. Two major commercial applications have emerged: recovery and recycle of hydrogen as in several industrial processes, and acid gas (carbon disulfide and hydrogen sulfide) removal from natural gas streams [2].

Electrodialysis

Electrodialysis (ED) differs significantly from the pressure-driven membrane processes in that an electrical force is used to drive the process. Only ions are transferred across the membrane barrier, and the membranes themselves are ion exchange membranes. Nevertheless, electrodialysis is a membrane process operating by the movement of materials through selective membranes and consequently is prone to the same kinds of problems as the pressure-driven processes such as boundary layer formation and membrane fouling [19].

The principle of electrodialysis is that electrical potential gradients make charged molecules diffuse in a medium at rates far greater than attainable by chemical potentials between two liquids, as in conventional dialysis. When a direct electric current is transmitted through a saline solution, most salts and minerals are dissolved in water as positively charged particles, cations and negatively charged particles, anions. The cations migrate toward the negative terminal, or cathode, and the anions toward the positive terminal, the anode. By adjusting the potential between the terminals the flow of ions transported between the plates can be varied. Additional control over the movement of the ions can be insured by placing membranes of cation or anion exchange material between the electrical plates. These sheets of cation-selective and anion-selective resins permit the passage of the respective ions in the solution. Under an applied d.c. field the cation and anions will collect on one side of each membrane through which they are specifically transported. Electrodialysis lends itself to the continuous-flow type of operations needed in industry. Multimembrane stacks can be built from alternatively spacing anionic- and cationic-selective membranes. Flow of solutions through specific compartments and appropriate recombination of transported ions permit desired enrichment of one stream and depletion of another [19].

Among the technical problems associated with the electrodialysis process, concentration-polarization is one of the most serious. This phenomenon adversely affects the operation of membranes and can even damage or destroy them. Polarization occurs when the movement of ions through the membrane is greater than the convective and diffusional movements of ions in the bulk solutions toward and away from the membrane. Along with a deleterious pH shift occurring at the membrane surface, polarization may cause solution contamination and sharply decrease energy efficiency. Commercial electrodialyzer incorporate turbulence promoters and limit current densities to avoid these effects. Other problems in practical applications include membrane scaling by inorganics in the feed solution and membrane fouling by organics. Efficient separation of suspended matter from the influent stream, by activated carbon absorption, can reduce or prevent such problems. Periodic flushing of membranes with acid solutions and/or detergent washing solutions is a conventional practice. An operational means of reducing the scaling and fouling problems consists of cyclical reversal cathodes and anodes along with interchanging the concentration and dilution streams [19].

Combination Electrodialysis and Ultrafiltration

One new technique being explored to utilize electromembrane processing concepts is combination electrodialysis/ultrafiltration. In a typical cheese whey concentration application, the process utilizes three membranes. These are a cation exchange selective membrane, an anion selective membrane, and an ultrafiltration membrane to retain proteins.

Transport depletion is similar to electrodialysis except that a neutral or non-ion selective membrane is used instead of an anion selective membrane. The special feature of this process is that the neutral membrane is less expensive and less subject to fouling than the anion exchange membranes. The economics and overall effectiveness of the process are similar to classic electrodialysis. However, production rates are usually a little lower and the electrical power consumption is slightly higher. The advantage of this process is lower membrane replacement cost. The disadvantage stems from the absence of ion selectivity of one of the membranes, limiting the potential for higher percentage demineralization. Transport depletion is less suitable at high demineralization or deacidification levels.

The develoment of bipolar membranes for electrodialysis processes has opened up a wide array of potential applications and warrants continued attention. The bipolar membrane is a cation-exchange membrane on one side and an anion-exchange membrane on the other side. There is a thin solution between the two sides of the membrane that results in a high resistance if the membranes are not fused. Water between the membranes dissociates and the bipolar membrane itself acts as an electrode. Bipolar membranes have been used to generate an acid and a base simultaneously from an acid/base salt; to regenerate sulfur dioxide absorber in flue gas desulfurization applications; for the conversion of poly ammonium salts into corresponding amines and acids; for production of carbon dioxide and pure sodium hydroxide from various sources of impure sodium salts; and for the conversion of hydroxylamine hydrochloride into hydroxylamine nitrate.

MECHANICAL METHODS

A number of separation methods are based on physical phenomena. The use of centrifugal forces or pressure forces, falls in this group.

Ultracentrifugation

The modern ultracentrifuge utilizes intense gravity forces (up to 400,000 g) generated by the centrifugal forces of a rapidly rotating rotor (up to 70,000 rpm). These high gravity forces are used to separate subcellular fractions such as protein, which, because they may be relatively close in mass, are difficult to separate by other means. The gravity forces due to rotation, causes sedimentation and differential separation of the heterogeneous particulates suspended in the solution. At completion of centrifugation, the large particles are found in a pellet at the bottom of the centrifuge vessel while small particles are still suspended in solution. Only partial separation is possible using differential centrifugation because the pellet zone is contaminated with other particle species since all particles will settle, although at different rates. To solve this problem, rate-zonal centrifugation using liquid density gradients, has been introduced resulting in higher resolution [19].

The amount of material which can be separated by rate-zonal centrifugation in a density gradient is severely limited. Other problems associated with rate-zonal centrifugation include the fact that sedimenting particles hit the wall (wall effect) of the centrifuge before they reach the bottom of the tube, and streaming in which the sample layer tends to break up into droplets which sediment through the gradient.

To provide for maximum sample sizes while minimizing the difficulties mentioned above, a hollow-bowl-shaped rotor was introduced; in this device, the interior is divided into compartments using radially arranged vertical septa. The septa serve to insure uniformity of acceleration and deceleration of the fluid in the rotor, preventing loss of separation resolution. Gradients and samples are introduced into the rotor while it is spinning, and recovery of the gradient with its separated zones is accomplished similarly. The gradient may be moved radially during rotation by pumping dense fluid to the rotor edge or light fluid to the rotor center. This enables combinations of rate and isopycnic separations. For example, cell membranes and mitochondria band isopycnically in the same layer of a sucrose gradient solution. They sediment at different rates, however, so the more slowly moving mitochondria may be unloaded with the sample layer while the more rapidly sedimenting cell membranes have banded in the sucrose gradient. While many particles in cell homogenates have sedimentation coefficients in the range of most viruses, few have the same sedimentation rate and banding density as viruses. Thus, this method may be used to separate these particles.

The possibility of moving the gradients during rotation permits large volumes of virus-containing fluids to be introduced into a small steep gradient, thereby sedimenting all the virus into a narrow band. By replacing the same layer many times, the virus particles from large volumes of sample may be recovered and simultaneously purified by isopycnic banding. The preparation of vaccines particularly has been aided by the development of continuous charging of the sample layer at high speed.

Actual commercial uses of ultracentrifugation include purification and separation of viruses, protein separation in the manufacture of cosmetics and enzymes, protein separation from human and animal serum, and the analysis of water samples for biomass, chemicals, and minerals [19].

Several problems have tended to limit the usefulness of the ultracentrifuge. Ultracentrifuge cells are subjected to large forces and have been prone to leaking. Rotors and bearings deteriorate with use, requiring that the ultracentrifuge be used at less than its rated maximum rotational speed. Large stresses and forces limit the useful lifetime of the ultracentrifuge. Ongoing research programs dealing with high-strength materials, oil-powered drives and high-pressure seals are attempting to alleviate these problems. They will have to be solved before the ultracentrifuge will be extensively utilized by industry. The most important factors holding back ultracentrifugation from extensive use in industry are its applicability to relatively low flow processes, and its energy and equipment intensiveness.

Nevertheless, the ultracentrifuge is being used in biotechnology as in the exemplary case described here [20]. In most large fermentation processes, a major concern is the removal of microorganisms and isolation of the metabolic products. In a few cases, such as production of single cell protein (especially yeast), the microorganisms themselves constitute the desirable end product. Centrifugal separators have been developed to effectively segregate the yeast from the fermentation broth. In the production of antibiotics, for example, a network of filaments (mycelia) at times makes filtration difficult. Various centrifugal separators can effectively remove the microorganisms without addition of other filtering aids. The decanter, solid-ejecting separator and nozzle separator are well suited for harvesting microorganisms. The main elements of the decanter are a rotating bowl supported at both ends and an internally arranged screw conveyor turning in the same direction as the bowl, but at a slightly lower speed. Bowl and screw are connected at one end by a planetary gear, which causes the difference in speed of rotation. The suspension to be separated is introduced through a feed tube passing through the hollow shaft of the bowl. The action of the angular acceleration throws the suspension against the wall of the bowl; the heavier component is deposited on the wall and the lighter liquid forms an inner layer. The solids are caught by the passing conveyor and fed toward one of the bowl ends and discharged. Solids-ejecting separators are disk-bowl machines that eject the solids intermittently during operation. A self-triggering device actuates the opening mechanism when the sludge space is filled up, thus making the machine fully automatic.

Harvesting of cells might become easier in a tissue culture system using fluorocarbon droplets instead of microscopic polymeric beads support. The droplets containing a surfactant are suspended in a culture medium to form an emulsion. A protein layer forms on the droplet and serves to anchor cells. Centrifugation can then be used to separate the culture into three layers: fluorocarbon, cells, and culture medium. The cells are then separated from the microcarriers by the action of trypsin. The technique appears promising for growth and purification of monoclonal antibodies and cell growth [21].

Continuous flow ultracentrifugation has been applied to the large scale purification of viruses, recovery of bacteria from dilute solutions, chloroplast, isolation, human plasma fractionation and the removal of microsomes [22]. The technique has proven reliable in spite of some sample leakage.

Cyclones are low cost centrifugal devices used in many chemical applications. They are simple devices with no moving parts. They are used for thickening ahead of centrifuges, degritting, counterculture washing, recovering crystals from solution. They can be made of a range of material and operated at elevated temperatures, high pressures and under corrosive and abrasive conditions.

Filtration

Filtration is a process for the separation of solids from liquid by use of a porous medium. Filter media includes woven fabrics, wire cloth and other porous mixtures. The two major mechanisms of filtration are cake and depth filtration. In the first case, a solid—the cake—is accumulated on a porous filter medium; in the second the solid is trapped within the medium using disposable cartridges or solid adsorbent. Filtration can be accomplished by mechanical action, the use of electric energy, or centrifugal forces. Cross flow filtration is actually based on molecular size. In all cases solids are separated from liquids. Polyelectrolyte flocculants, synthetic fibers and membranes, and endless belt filters have enlarged the domain of applicability of cake filtration. Batch pressure and continuous pressure filters are commonly used. Vacuum filter systems (batch and continuous) are available. Cartridge filtering is usually used for classification rather than product recovery. An electric field may be imposed on a suspension to augment filtration.

Separation of solid aggregates of different sizes poses formidable problems. Commercially available filters are often unable to discriminate by size, which results in concentrating both substances rather than passing one through the filter with the liquid. This problem is particularly important in the production of biopolymers such as those used in enhanced oil recovery. During conventional biopolymer separation, alcohol is used to precipitate a by-product. This step contributes as much as 40% of the total production cost. The criterion of good separation is the production of a solution of the desired viscosity (i.e., a viscosity that does not unacceptably plug oil well formations) without loss of substantial fractions of the biopolymer in the process. The method described below is a laboratory-scale technique ultimately to be used in field production of the biopolymer, scleroglucan, followed by the wet separation of scleroglucan from the fermentation broth [23]. *Sclerotium solfsii* is grown in a fermenter sparged by air. Mechanical agitation and ambient temperature are maintained. The resultant broth is passed through a variety of filtering equipment (e.g., axial filters and microscreens/microstrainers) to separate scleroglucan particles. In this case, an axial filter where a membrane is wrapped around a rotor spun in a chamber, and into which feed is introduced under pressure. The rotor is perforated, and passages are provided for filtrate to exit through the axis. Filtration is carried out at 200 psig (13.6 bars) and at 200 rpm, corresponding to about 11 ft/sec (335 cm/sec). These filters are developed to eliminate the necessity for a precipitation step during biopolymer separation. It has been demonstrated that capital cost and power requirements using microscreening at a 100-kg/day biopolymer plant are approximately $80,000 and 6 kW, respectively. Biopolymer separation using microscreens and axial filters is less costly and more energy-efficient than separation using diatomaceous earth filters or centrifugation. Microscreens and microstrainers made of plastic and of stainless steel and having different apertures have been applied to the removal of biomass from fermentation broth [23].

LIQUID-SOLID-GAS INTERACTION METHODS

A number of separation techniques are based on specific interactions between liquids, solids and gases.

Absorption

This is a physical process that involves transferring one or more constituents from a gas phase to a liquid phase. Typically the lean solvent enters an absorber at the top and flows downward in a countercurrent mode making contact with the rising chemically laden vapor stream. Through mixing and contact in plates and trays, the solute is transferred from the gas to the liquid solvent.

The solvent must be carefully selected for each application. Ideally, the solvent is nonvolatile, inexpensive, noncorrosive or flammable, stable, nonviscous and nonforming, and with a great affinity for the species of interest. Under proper conditions, high recovery is achieved.

Adsorption

The use of carbon for filtration was originally discovered by the ancient Egyptians. The quality of the carbon has improved since, but the principle remains the same. All solids will adsorb fluids or gas molecules on their surface. Porous substances will adsorb more because of their extended surface. Carbon is used because of its high porosity (a pound of carbon can have up to 6 million square feet of surface) and nonpolar characteristics (which allow it to adsorb organic molecules). Polar adsorbants such as activated alumina and silica gel adsorb inorganic molecules only.

Activated carbon may be made from nearly every organic material by carbonizing. Among the most common materials are wood, coal, nut shells, and petroleum residues. Various processing steps are required to assure that the raw material will be converted to activated carbon. The last step in the activation process consists of heating in a controlled oxidizing atmosphere to produce the large surface area desired.

There are various grades of activated carbon which result from various methods of preparation; the different grades will have differing properties for use in different applications. Fine pore size materials are applicable to materials with small molecules while coarse pore sizes are used for trapping larger molecules.

Activated carbon is generally supplied in the form of pellets of varying sizes and properties to match specific applications. For certain applications, the activated carbon can be supplied in molded preformed shapes. In these cases, the carbon is bonded with a water insoluble agent which does not substantially interfere with the adsorption process. In some applications, the carbon is supplied in large dimensionally stable shapes which can serve as their own containers, thereby eliminating the cost of the container.

Activated carbon filters may be used to recover solvents including acetone, benzene, cyclohexane, dichloromethane, ethanol, ethyl acetate, ethyl benzene, freons, isopropanol, methanol, methyl ethyl ketone, methyl isobutyl ketone, naphtha, tetrahydrofuran, toluene, and xylene.

After a period of operation, the filter will become ineffective and it will then require regeneration. To regenerate it, the filter must be taken out of operation and heated. The heating reevaporates (desorbs) the adsorbed vapors and these can be recovered or flared off, depending on the economics of the process. The heating is usually performed by the use of steam.

Activated carbon adsorption systems are very efficient. Efficiencies of 99% vapor removal from the steam are quite common, with total system vapor recovery exceeding 90%. After a long period of operation, normal regeneration becomes ineffective due to the presence of high boiling or polymerized materials and reactivation becomes necessary. Reactivation is performed on a custom basis (as it depends on the foreign materials present), and in general consists of heating the carbon under a controlled atmosphere to a temperature of 900 °C.

Ion exchange is a reversible process. Ions are exchanged between a liquid and a solid phase. Resins with specific ion active sites are the solid phase. Such techniques for sugar separation and purification (glucose-fructose, sorbitol, mannitol) are commonplace. Weak acid ion exchange resins are used in the isolation and purification of antibiotics.

Inorganic ion exchangers include mineral zeolites and clay. Organic ion exchangers include weak acid cation exchange resin primarily based on acrylic and methacrylic acid cross linked with a difunctional monomer. Strong acid resins are sulfonated copolymers of styrene and

DVB. Anion exchange resins and acid absorbers are based on primary, secondary and tertiary amine functionality. Other functional groups are used for specific applications.

Adsorption is an exothermic process. The heat generated during the process is usually carried out of the bed. Now comes an energy efficient adsorption cycle making use of this heat. The method has been used to break down water organic azeotropes and remove large amounts of water. The system operates in a manner such that a substantial part of heat generated during adsorption is stored, and then used during the desorption step, hence reducing the volume and temperature of the purge gas [24].

Inorganic salts such as ammonium sulphate are used in large scale enzyme purification processes. The major disadvantage is the long contact times required. Methanol, n-propanol, and acetone have been used as precipitation agents. The major disadvantage is the large energy consumption associated with the solvent recovery step. A new technique avoids both problems. It is based on counter current adsorption. The method has been applied to separate cellulase from cellulose-sugar mixtures. The removal of the enzyme from the hydrolysate is achieved by countercurrent contacting with fresh cellulose. Mixing cellulose with its substrate results in almost immediate absorption of the enzyme. The enzyme is slowly released as cellulose is solubilized at 25–50 °C and pH 4.0–5.0 [25].

Fuel-grade ethanol is produced by fermentation of waste biomass where the final concentration of the product is typically 90% ethanol and 10% water. To use ethanol as a fuel, one must obtain a 99% solution. Distillation, which is costly and energy-intensive, is the most commonly used process; therefore, the cost of the purification step has a significant effect on the ultimate cost of the fuel-grade ethanol. The experimental system described here is a bench-scale continuous column adsorption process used to selectively adsorb ethanol on hydrophobic sorbents followed by desorption carried out with preheated nitrogen [75 °C(167 °F)] to recover ethanol vapor. The results of early tests with a copolymer resin (styrenedivinylbenzene) and a proprietary molecular sieve indicate that, although the molecular sieve yields purer ethanol, neither has sufficient selectivity to make the process highly feasible. Further studies have been recommended including alternative materials for the molecular sieve and alternative desorption processes. Water, as well as ethanol, is sorbed onto the sorbent surface, indicating that selectivity is not adequate. Sorbent materials tend to erode under flow conditions. Additional work is necessary to design an effective desorption apparatus. Sorption may represent a low-cost alternative to the energy-intensive process of distillation [26].

Affinity precipitation is a procedure whereas water soluble polymer bearing appropriate ligand groups are added to a broth for stepwise removal of products of interest. The polymers contain precipitation groups which permit quantitative precipitation of the polymer bearing the products by pH changes on the addition of a salt. The technique has been successfully applied to the purification of trypsin from beef pancreas. The major advantages are specificity, high overall recovery yield, speed, low cost, application to large volumes, and the possibility to repeatedly apply the technique for sequential removal of products. The technique should find many new applications in the future [27].

Solvent Extraction

Liquid-liquid extraction depends on the transfer of a solute from one liquid phase to another formed by two immiscible solvents in contact with each other. This is an equilibrium phenomena of great versatility because of the enormous range of solvents available today. It is common for solvent extraction to incorporate a chemical reaction between the solute to be extracted and a reactant dissolved in the solvent. The technique is especially applicable to heat labile products that cannot be separated by thermal methods. Cross current and counter current extraction schemes are used in a continuous fashion in the industry. Improvements in multistage and differential contactors have given a broad range of application to the technique.

Commercial extractors include spray columns easy to operate, packed columns with high efficiency and perforated-plate columns for stagewise operations. Mixer-settlers of high capacity are used commercially. Centrifugal extractors accelerate phase separation by the use of centrifugal force and achieve minimum residence time. The industrial applications are many in the petrochemical, food and pharmaceutical industries. Antibiotics (penicillin, streptomycin) and vitamins (A,B,C,D, E) are extracted this way.

Liquid-liquid extraction, or leaching, is a very old technique. The operation depends on the solubility of the material to be extracted or the ability of the solvent to react with the solid material in order to produce a soluble reactant. This technique is used extensively in the mineral ore extraction industry. It is also in use in the extraction of sugar from sugar beets, vegetable oils from oilseeds, soluble coffee from coffee beans, flavors and essences from botanical materials.

Liquid-liquid fractionation is often used for protein separation. Ammonium sulfate, alcohol, acetone and polyethylene glycol are the most often used fractionation agents. Temperature, because of its effect on solubility, is a key control parameter. Two phase aqueous partition systems have been used to differentiate proteins from cell debris, for enzyme purification, for the removal of nucleic acids and other interfering substances [28]. Disk stack separators and nozzle separators are quite efficient in enzymes separation (high yield) and use a minimum of energy in a rapid fashion.

In a process developed by the Georgia Institute of Technology and commercialized by Dynes Holding Co. (Atlanta, GA), the ethanol solution is continuously drawn off from a conventional fermenter. The solution contacts a solvent in a countercurrent liquid/liquid extraction column. Solvents such as higher molecular weight alcohols, organophosphates and paraffins have been tested. The concept promises to be energy efficient and to have a major impact on the cost of ethanol.

Supercritical Fluid Extraction

The specialty chemicals and the biotechnology industries need an extraction process which can remove some highly volatile substances from the chemical mixtures in order to make a product with the desired formulation. To satisfy this need, some laboratory scale experiments have been successfully conducted with the help of supercritical CO_2. This process has been tried on compounds which differ with respect to molecular weight and the number and nature of their functional groups (ranging from nonpolar hydrocarbons to strongly polar substances) [29–32].

This discussion of supercritical solution is centered on the characteristics of carbon dioxide and its behavior as a supercritical solvent. Other solvents such as pentane, toluene, ethane and inert gases, have also been used. The phase diagram of carbon dioxide shows the equilibrium pressures and temperatures between gaseous liquid and solid carbon dioxide.

The primary region of concern is shown in the upper right-hand side of the figure where the CO_2 reaches its critical temperature 304.2 °K (31.1 °C) and critical pressure 73.86 bars. The density of the carbon dioxide at the critical point is 0.468 g/cm³. In the supercritical region, carbon dioxide exists as a single fluid completely filling the vessel without showing a meniscus between liquid and gas. CO_2 is a very poor solvent. As pressure is increased, its density increases and its extractive power improves substantially.

The addition of a soluble substance (solute) to the carbon dioxide will change the conditions for the formation of the supercritical region. Change in conditions are required to obtain supercritical solutions for substances of different molecular weights and the presence of polar groups which can interact with the carbon dioxide. For linear hydrocar-

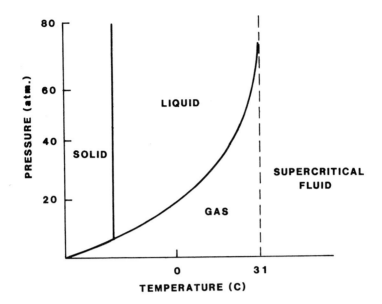

bons, the formation of a supercritical solution phase tends toward higher temperatures and pressures as the molecular weight (molecular size) increases. The presence of a polar functional group (i.e., hydroxyl group), also increases the pressure and temperature for critical solution formation when compared with the parent hydrocarbon. The presence of a second polar group requires higher temperatures and pressures for the formation of critical solutions. Water, which has a low molecular weight, undergoes chemical reaction with carbon dioxide to form carbonic acid. This, and the higher critical temperature and pressure of water, adds to the temperature and pressure requirements for forming a supercritical solution of two substances.

This sensitivity of critical solution formation to the solute molecular weight, polarity, spatial configuration (i.e., molecular shape), and extent of chemical bonding of solutes and solvents, among other factors, make it necessary to determine the phase diagrams for the systems of interest. The addition of a second or more solutes adds to the complexity of the system, and where several solutes may be involved, the relationships must be determined experimentally.

Using compressed gas as solvent for extraction is becoming increasingly interesting. It has been used commercially to remove caffeine from green coffee, to extract flavoring ingredients from hops, and for botanical extractions.

Conventional hop extraction generally employs dichloromethane which has to be evaporated after the hop resins have been extracted. The resulting extract is a pasty, dark-green to black-green mass which is not permitted to contain more than 2.2% solvent residue (CH_2Cl_2). Under the first case [33], to produce hop extract with supercritial CO_2, commercial hop pellets are subjected to pressure range of approximately 80 to 300 atmospheres at temperatures of 35 to 80°C. An olive green, pasty extract with an intensive aroma of hops is obtained. The pellets disintegrate into a powder which can easily be shaken out of the extraction vessel. Extract separation by releasing the pressure in several stages is currently being investigated. In the second case [34], the entire soft resin and the essential oils of the hops, but less than 100% of the hard resin fraction can be extracted by use of extraction pressures of from 100 to 220 atmospheres gauge.

Evaluation of the results to date shows that a wide variety of types of substances can be extracted with supercritical CO_2 in the lower pressure range alone. Extractability falls sharply in the pressure range up to 400 bars, particularly following the introduction of polar functional groups. The findings can be summarized as follows [29]:

- Hydrocarbons and other typically lipophilic organic compounds of relatively low polarity (e.g., esters, ethers, lactones, and epoxides) can be extracted in the lower pressure range of 70 to 100 bar.
- The introduction of strongly polar functional groups (e.g., —OH, —COOH) makes the extraction more difficult. In the range of benzene derivatives, substances with three phenoic hydroxyls are still capable of extraction.

The observation that an increase in temperature at constant pressure is accompanied by a decrease in density and hence improved ability to transport material has formed the basis of the application of supercritical CO_2 to the separation of mixtures of high boiling point materials which are not amenable to fractional distillation under normal conditions [35].

In the specialty chemicals industry, supercritical CO_2 extraction is of increasing interest [29]:

- Many expensive organic compounds (used as raw material for formulation of specialty chemicals) are lost to the waste stream resulting from the production process. CO_2 (in its supercritical state) is considered to be a very effective solvent to recover these compounds.
- Because it is a good solvent to recover organics, it is an effective technology for treatment of effluents from chemical production facilities.

The use of supercritical CO_2 as a unit operation is energy efficient. In the production of ethanol, for example, it is possible to concentrate a gallon with a countercurrent of supercritical CO_2 using just half the energy it takes to distill the same amount (6 kWh) in most modern plants from the fermented mash [36]. Supercritical extraction for any application is energy efficient because of the simple fact that supercritical separations are carried out at temperatures that are moderate by chemical process standards and since vaporizing and condensing CO_2 consume little energy [29].

Supercritical extraction is a solvent process which, when developed, can replace some distillation processes in various industries. In chemical and petroleum refining industries it can result in substantial energy saving because the solvent processes, by their very nature, are less energy intensive. These two industries use 3% of the total U.S. energy required for industry for their distillation processes [37].

This developing technology offers a viable alternative to the conventional, mostly energy-intensive, chemical processes. It is evident that the economics of the technology depend on the particular application. If the technology is applied to commodity chemicals, for example, it will not be very economical because the typical cost of supercritical extraction is estimated at 5 to 10 cents (U.S. currency) per pound (0.45 kg) of material treated, while most of the commodity chemicals are themselves in the 5 to 20 cents range. It may be economical when applied to specialty chemicals which have a much higher value [29].

The above holds true for the initial capital costs involved in building a commercial plant. These could be substantially higher for industries (such as food industry) because at 5,000 psi (351.5 kg per square centimeter) the processes cannot be carried out by the equipment currently in use in these industries. They need to install pumps and plumbing able to withstand high pressure conditions [36,37].

Chromatography

Chromatography is an extraction process using selective absorbents. The affinity absorbent is placed in contact with a solution containing several substances, including the species to be isolated. The ligate is attached specifically to the ligand. The non-binding species are washed up. The ligate is recovered by elution. The ligand can be a polymeric substrate, an enzyme, an antibody, an antigen, a polysaccharide, an inhibitor, a cofactor, a prostetic group, or nucleic acid.

Chromatography is one of the most common separation techniques for analytical and preparative work. Rapid progress in technology has given rise to a bewildering assortment of concepts, support material, mobile phases, columns, and peripheral equipment.

The most common method of using affinity sorbent chromatography is a packed column. High efficiency and ease of automation are important advantages; low throughout because of bed clogging is an always present problem. Multi-sequence columns arrangements are attractive for isolating several species simultaneously. A number of batch operations are frequently employed to alleviate the disadvantages of packed columns. The tea bag method involves inserting the sorbent into porous bags and immersing them into the solution. By having several bags with different sorbents, it is possible to isolate several species in one operation. The continuous belt technique involves incorporating the ligand into a meshed fabric shaped into a continuous belt. The belt in the form of an endless loop is transported through a sequence of tanks including the sample solution, rinse bath, recovery solution and regeneration bath.

Chromatography for protein purification takes many forms: size exclusion [38], ion exchange [39], hydrophobic and affinity chromatography. Other chromatographic techniques of great interest in preparative biotechnology include: metal ion liquid chromatography [40], reversed phase chromatography [41], low pressure liquid chromatography [41], the mono bed fast protein liquid chromatography [43], and foam chromatography based on surfactants action [44].

Liquid chromatography uses soft bed packing material and as such cannot be subject to high operating pressures and fast flow rates. In order to increase the speed of chromatographic separation, rigid and semi-rigid packing materials are used. This way high peformance liquid chromatography has been scaled up to the gram-kilogram level of separation for small polypeptides. Wide pore columns have been used with great success in separating leukocyte interferons from several species at the milligram level. Efficient liquid chromatography is determined by column length, particle size and packing quality. Other determining factors include mobile phase velocity and viscosity and temperature. Modern liquid chromatographs are smaller, use less solvent and are more rapid. These progresses are achieved by trade off among the variables mentioned above [45]. Full automation of the process is providing finer control of the process [46,47].

Aqueous gel filtration chromatography (GFC), although available for many years for protein and enzymes purification and preparation based on dextran, agarose and polyacrylamide is inexpensive and easy to use but it suffers from many drawbacks. Conventional gels cannot tolerate high pressures or high flow rates. Extraordinary long separation time is involved. The dextran matrix cannot tolerate extremes of salt, pH, and organic solvents. Most of these problems have been solved with the advent of inexpensive, small size, porous, semi-rigid spherical gels synthetized from hydrophilic vinyl polymers [48]. The gels have proven well suited for separation, purification, and fractionation of proteins, enzymes, nucleic acids, oligosaccharides, and many other biochemical materials. The gels performed well in the pH range of 1 to 14. They are thermally stable (sterilization at 120 °C is possible). They are highly resistant to microbial attack. They can stand pressure up to 100 psi. They have been applied to protein separation, with good retention of activity, from hundreds of millions molecular weight. They are ideally suited for biotechnology applications.

The unique feature and advantage of countercurrent chromatography (CCG) is its operation without a solid support often incriminated in sample loss and chemical degradations. The method is based on the observation that immiscible liquids in coiled tubes could be segmented and made to undergo countercurrent flow. Phase separation takes place in a gravitational field but can be enhanced by rotating the column in a centrifugal field. The major advantages of CCG include no need for support material, a wide choice of two-phase solvent systems, less troublesome emulsion, shorter separation time, solvent conservation, improved efficiency, quantitative recovery, avoidance of product modification and rearrangement and compact arrangement. It is expected that CCG will be competitive in the future with HPLC for a wide variety of natural products. This method has great potential for the rapid separaton of cells and macromolecules [49,50].

The success of high pressure liquid chromatography (HPLC) hinges on the continuing development of efficient microparticulate supports, a stable stationary phase with a broad spectrum of selective properties and the availability of peripheral equipment capable of delivering solvents at high pressure and flow rates. HPLC offers advantages in resolution, speed and ease of quantitative sample recovery [39]. A recently announced protein purification system features a 30 cm in diameter and 3 meter high column. A hydraulically driven piston forces the fluid through the packing material. The efficiency level is equivalent to 11,000 theoretical plates per meter. The capacity is 1Kg/hr and the flow is 500 l/hrs at a pressure of 500 bars.

Reversed-phase chromatography is based on a nonpolar stationary phase, a porous microparticulate chemically bounded alkyl silica and a polar mobile phase. Separation is based on hydrophobic contacts between the molecule of interest and the stationary phase. Excellent resolution and separation can be achieved. High selectivity and short separation time is emphasized. Most polypeptides and protein bind strongly to alkylsilica and must be specifically eluted. Today some 65% of all chromatography is conducted using the reversed phase technique [45]. Multisolvent chromatography is rapidly becoming the norm.

Ion exchange chromatography of polypeptides and proteins is not extensive. The technique seeks to discriminate between molecules by an ion exchange process based on the ionic character of the proteins. Preparative separation of hormones and enzymes yields biological activity greater than 90%.

High performance size exclusion chromatography (HPSEC) of proteins on surface modified silicas and hydrophilic organic polymers has achieved success. Exploiting the ionic or hydrophobic properties of the support material, a weak mobile phase achieves high recovery of protein mass and biological activity in rapid elution times. The technique is especially applicable to labile enzymes unfavorably treated by ion exchange or reverse phased columns. The technique is not as successful with small peptides (1,000–10,000 MW) and can handle only modest load.

Affinity or immunosorbent chromatography is based on immobilizing an enzyme on a column. When a protein with impurities is passed on this column, the enzyme of interest is covalently bound to the immobilized protein. The desired protein is then recovered by washing the column with an appropriate solvent or buffer. Such techniques have ready to move from the laboratory to the large scale production scale. An example is the purification and concentration of urokinase from urine using a monoclonal antibody immobilized on a packed column. Affinity columns have been applied to the separation of bovine serum albumine, the plasminogen activating enzyme urokinase, and galactosidase. A requirement for affinity separation methods is for the adsorbent to function with crude enzyme liquids or in the presence of high cell debris. Much success has been achieved with non porous particles [51].

Antigen antibody reaction in repetitive columns offers good possibilities for isolating specific protein in good yield. It is today possible to raise antibodies for any protein extending tremendously the range of applicability of immunoadsorption methods [52]. Monoclonal antibodies against alpha interferon have been used to concentrate human interferon [53].

Cell harvesting is an important step in biotechnology operations. Two techniques are worth mentioning. The first is a cell affinity chromatography by immobilized ligands to insoluble matrices through cleavable mercury-sulfur bonds. Mouse lymphocytes and sheep red blood cells have been successfully separated [54]. The second used liquid-phase positive immunoselection [55].

THERMAL METHODS

Heat as a driving force for dewatering and concentration is probably the oldest separation and purification method.

Distillation

Distillation is a separation process that takes advantage of the difference in boiling points of liquids in a number of vaporization and condensation steps. As an example, in the brewery industry, a significant amount of liquid effluent needs to be treated for reduction of BOD. The costs for the treatment of brewery effluents are high, and those for treating effluent containing residual alcohol are likely to be more expensive. Currently available treatment methods do not produce a salable by-product, which could aid in offsetting the effluent treatment costs. Distillation can recover a large amount of valuable ethanol from waste brewery effluents, thus offering a salable by-product as well as reducing BOD levels. Brewery effluent contains a mixture of suspended solids, soluble solids, ethyl alcohol, water and small quantities of other volatiles. Since the ethyl alcohol contributes significantly to the BOD of the effluent, and since ethyl alcohol is a valuable by-product in a concentrated form, it is important to remove this effluent, purify it and produce a salable liquid that will help to offset the costs of treatment. The alcohol content of the brewery effluent (especially from distillation) ranges 2–4% (v/v) together with minor amounts of other volatiles such as aldehydes.

These vaporization and condensation steps consume vast amounts of energy, close to 3% (2 × 10^{15} Btu) of all U.S. energy consumption [56]. Several energy conservation techniques (e.g., heat exchanges, air preheaters) can be used during distillation, however, vapor recompression offers a method for more efficient use of heat energy, typically reducing energy input to the distillation tower between 10 and 15% [57].

In the face of rising energy costs, it is necessary to modify or retrofit distillation plants to reduce energy consumption. This is true in biotechnology applications where distillation is an option for purification. Several methods of economizing energy in a distillation plant are possible; one of the most effective methods is energy recovery. The three main methods for recovering energy include the multiple-effect method, indirect vapor recompression and direct vapor recompression. Direct vapor recompression is the most energy-efficient choice.

The key operational variables in vapor recompression installation include the pressure difference between the top and the bottom of the distillation tower, the absolute pressure level of the tower (which affects both the relative volatility and the compression ratio), and the log mean temperature difference [57]. A vapor compression system can be used to reboil the contents of one or more adjacent distillation towers to minimize energy requirements and to maximize material and waste heat reuse. Energy demand in conventional process can be improved using vapor recompression by the use of waste energy to replace raw energy, and by providing mechanically aided (i.e., compressed fluid) heat in addition to direct use of waste water.

With some process modification, distillation systems can be retrofitted to improve separation of close boiling components. In a typical system, overhead vapors pass from the column to a compressor drum where they are compressed to saturation temperature. They are then desuperheated by exchange with cooling water. Since compression of vapors results in superheating, a heat exchanger is required in addition to the reboiler. The condensed vapors flow to the reflux drum from the reboiler (condenser); pressure is greater in the reflux drum than the column pressure removing the need for a reflux pump. Reflux is subcooled by exchange with pumped column bottoms and returned to the column while the propylene is sent to storage. The operation results in a decrease in cooling water requirements and an elimination of the steam requirement but at the same time increases the need for energy in the form of electricity.

The recovery of high-boiling fractions from mixtures containing a large proportion of low-boiling fractions is an expensive process. The conventional method of separation is by fractional distillation. The steam consumption, for a mixture containing 10% (by weight) of less volatile components and a reflux ratio of 1, is about 20 tons per tone of the less-volatile component. By use of vapor recompression as an integral part of the rectification, steam consumption is reduced. The column overhead containing pure, more-volatile components is allowed to flow into the compressor and, before returning to the column reboiler (condenser), the superheated vapor is cooled to its saturation point by the injection of condensed steam. The less-volatile component, removed from the bottom of the first column, is vaporized in a pre-evaporator and fed into the second column. The top vapor in this second column contains the less-volatile component which must be recycled to the first column. As the quantity of the less-volatile component in the column rises, the differences between the bottom and top temperatures increases and, with it, the consumption of energy for compressing the vapors is also greatly increased. The costs of steam and electricity determine whether the costs of recovering less-volatile comonents can be reduced by the vapor recompression system [59].

A recent improvement to distillation is "paradistillation." The new approach split the vapor into two or more parts. As liquid falls through the column, half-moon trays force it to contact one vapor part, then another, alternatively. The paradistillation process gives 33% more theoretical plates than the traditional distillation [59].

Evaporation

Evaporators differ from conventional dryers in that the degree of dryness obtained in an evaporator is much less than that obtained in a dryer. Evaporators are particularly useful in those applications where it is not possible or required to reduce to very low level the moisture content of the product because the material is heat sensitive, does not readily lend itself to processing in a heat exchanger due to its viscous properties, or because of chemical constituents that exhibit fouling or foaming tendencies. There are several types of evaporators [60]:

Thin-Film Evaporators

Thin-film evaporators rely on mechanical blades that spread the process fluid across the heated surface of a large tube. The liquid or the slurry forms a thin film or annular ring of product from the feed nozzle to the product outlet nozzle. Volatiles driven off from the product rise counter-current to the descending liquid film and are removed at the top of the vaporizer. Product inventory or hold-up is very minimal, typically about one-half pound of material per square foot of heat transfer surface (2.44 Kg/m²).

Thin film evaporators have been in operation for about 40 years. Of the two most common types, vertical evaporators are by far the most used. This is due to the fact that vertical evaporators are far more versatile than horizontal ones. Vertical evaporators can process thick slurries or dilute solutions, with the same degree of ease. Whereas horizontal evaporators are restricted to material with viscosities in excess of one million centipoise.

Advantages associated with thin-film evaporators are: large heating surface, low inventory retention, small space requirements, and their suitability for processing heat sensitive materials. Disadvantages associated with these systems are: unsuitability for salting or severely scaling liquids, and unsuitability for processing liquids with suspended solids [60].

Multiple Effect Evaporators

In multiple effect evaporators, the material to be dried is processed in succeeding stages, each stage utilizing the hot exhaust gases and operating at a lower temperature than the preceding stage. Because of this feature, multiple stage evaporators are more efficient than single stage evaporators. In single effect evaporators, heat released by the condensing steam or by hot air is transferred to an aqueous solution. The solution absorbs heat and part of the water in the solution is evaporated causing the remaining solution to become richer in solute. The vapor is then discharged to a barometric or surface condenser where it releases its latent heat to cooling water [60].

Advantages associated with multiple evaporation are: low maintenance costs, reduced steam requirements, short residence time, ability to process a great range of materials, better drying performance than single effect evaporators. Disadvantages associated with these dryers are: high capital cost, in order to operate the vapors from the boiling liquors must be relatively low in impurities that may foul the vapor side of the heater exchanger.

Vapor Recompresson Evaporator

Vapor recompression evaporation differs from the other evaporation techniques in the way the steam is used. In this method, live steam is combined with the vapors combining from the solution being processed. At present, there are two methods of vapors recompression: thermal vapor recompression (TVR) and mechanical vapor recompression (MVR). The two differ in the manner in which the vapors are recycled and in the amounts which are utilized [58,60].

Evaporation is a unit operation with a high energy requirement. It involves the use of electrical energy for circulation and pumping as well as use of heat energy. These energy requirements can be minimized by the use of mechanical vapor recompression (MVR) in an evaporation cycle. Considerable savings in steam requirements can be achieved if, instead of using first stage vapor to heat a subsequent stage as in multiple effects evaporators, the vapor is mechanically compressed through a sufficient pressure range to be used as the heating medium in the stage where it is generated [61]. Reasons for using the vapor recompression system in evaporation are [62,63]:

- lower operating costs than any other type of evaporator;
- all evaporation takes place at one temperature which can be selected for optimum process considerations;
- no cooling water is required and any excess heat available is at the highest temperature in the system.

Mechanical recompression is most practical for low temperature differences and low boiling-point elevations. The evaporator components include a vapor head, a heating element, vapor piping, circulating piping, a circulating pump, and a compressor. The compressor raises the evaporator vapors to a higher energy level and reuses them in the heating element. The boiled-off vapors are compressed and used as the heating medium on the condensing steam side. In general, the vapor recompression cycle is estimated to require between 4 to 12 kWh per 1,000 pounds of product evaporated [62]. The operation of this evaporator takes advantage of the fact that it takes less energy to compress and recirculate the waste vapors to higher energy levels than it takes to heat water vapor to the same energy level [58,60].

Another type of vapor recompression used during evaporation is thermal vapor recompression (TVR). During thermal recompression, a compressor is utilized to reduce the heat load in the evaporator. A fraction of the overhead vapor is transported and compressed to a higher pressure and temperature with a high-pressure source of steam. Thermal recompression involves the compression of vapor given off from a single-effect evaporator to a higher pressure and temperature for use as the heating medium for the same evaporator. It is now possible to apply this principle to many industrial applications as a result of better compressor design, i.e., use of corrosion-free hardware requiring little maintenance.

The majority of large-scale evaporation operations that use multiple effect evaporators involve the removal of water which has a high latent heat of vaporization. This heat is absorbed into a cooling water system and is subsequently lost to the process. The ideal evaporation system is one in which all the heat in the vapor, exhausted from the evaporator, is re-cycled and reused in the system without change of state [64]. Vapor recompression evaporators are designed to approach this idea. Vapor recompression is best employed when evaporating large quantities of water from solutions which initially are rather dilute and which do not result in particularly viscous products or give rise to high boiling point elevations. Vapor recompression can potentially be used in the food processing industry to concentrate whey, juice, sugar, corn syrup, and corn steep liquor [60].

Advantages associated with TVR evaporators are: much lower steam requirements, low installation costs, increases the capacity of the equipment, reliability of mechanical performance, low maintenance costs. Advantages associated with MVR are: much lower steam requirements, increases the capacity of the equipment, no cooling water requirements, lesser space requirements than similar capacity equipment.

Disadvantages associated with TVR evaporators are: unsuitable for use in situations in which the boiling point rise is high, requires vapors which are low in impurities which may plug the steam jet. Disadvantages associated with MVR systems are: high capital costs, high maintenance costs, high power costs, requires vapors which are very low in impurities that may foul the compressor.

Drying Systems

Drying of solid is a common unit operation. The process is made difficult by the several forms taken by the liquid. Liquids that wet surfaces, liquid that occupies interstices in a solid, and liquid of hydration more tightly bound to molecules. Many industries require drying operations in the manufacture of their products. Since the materials to be dried differ greatly in their physical characteristics and degree of dryness required, the equipment involved takes on many forms [60,65,66].

In direct heat dryers, heat is applied directly to wet solid or liquid materials by the heating medium, usually a hot gas. The hot gas also acts as the moisture removing agent by carrying away the vapors removed from the material. In indirect heat dryers, heat is applied to the wet solid or liquid material by conduction from the heating medium by means of heat exchangers. In this type of dryer, air or gas flow, if used at all, serves only as the vapor removing agent. In the air-suspended systems, drying is accomplished much the same way as in direct drying systems. The particles to be dried are suspended and violently agitated in a stream of hot gas. Because of their ability to suspend the material to be dried, air suspended systems have shorter residence times than the other systems. However, the range of material that can be processed is limited to those which can be suspended in a gas stream.

Air-Suspended Systems

Direct drying systems rely on the bulk heat and mass properties of the material being processed. Air-suspended systems, because of the turbulent flow that exists inside the drying chamber, rely on the microscopic heat and mass transfer properties. In this system the rate of moisture removal is directly proportional to the:

- particle diameter;
- temeprature difference between the particle and drying gas;
- mass velocity of the drying gas;
- film coefficient for the heat transfer for the drying gas; and
- pressure.

There are three types of dryers in the air-suspended system. These are flash, spray, and fluidized-bed.

The flash dryer is merely an air conveyor into which heated air and the material to be dried are introduced sequentially. Drying time ranges from less than one second to about 10 seconds. In this type of dryer, particulate solids are introduced by a conveyor into a very fast moving hot gas stream. Normal air velocities are in the range of 4,000 to 6,000 ft/min (1219 to 1829 m/sec). The processed solids are usually separated from the gas phase in a cyclone [60]. Drying is very fast because the factors governing the rate of drying are optimized. The material is dispersed in the gas stream thus maximizing the surface area exposed to the gas. High inlet-gas temperature is used, because exposure time is short and the material remains in the wet-bulb temperature due to the rapid evaporation of the water. This gives a large temperature difference. Maximum agitation results from the turbulence due to high gas velocities. Advantages associated with flash dryers are: low capital cost; short residence time which avoids decomposition of heat sensitive material; conveying, milling and product recycle can be carried out simultaneously with the drying operaton; and low space requirements. Disadvantages associated with these systems are: that they do not remove occluded moisture; they are unsuitable for highly abrasive materials or large crystals that must not be broken; and they are unsuitable for materials with moisture content over 80%.

The fluid bed dryer is characterized by the moderate conditions under which it operates. Operating temperatures at the bed itself are low compared to flash and spray dryers. Air flow is such that it will cause the solids to remain suspended above the distributor plate. Because each particle is surrounded by gas, handling is gentle and little attrition occurs. Advantages associated with fluid-bed dryers are: close temperature control; retention time is reasonable, occluded moisture is effectively removed; simultaneous drying and size-classifying may be done; floor space requirements are small. Disadvantages associated with these dryers are: temperature of the distributor plate is high and may cause materials to stick to it; variations in particle size give variable dryer performance [67].

A spray is a liquid dispersed as droplets in a gas. The drops are formed during an atomization process in which a liquid column or sheet is broken up mechanically via rotation or vibration. The atomizers are either centrifugal pressure nozzles, solid cone nozzle or fan spray nozzles. Spray drying is widely used in drying products: coffee, tea, starch, pharmaceuticals, soaps, detergents and pigments. In spray dryers, the feed is atomized prior to being introduced into the air stream. The portion of the duct where the feed is introduced is enlarged to give the atomized particles time to dry before they contact the chamber walls.

The liquid feed may be atomized to a spray by a rotating disk, a high pressure nozzle or a two-fluid nozzle. As the energy input to the atomizer is increased, the average particle size and the particle size distribution will decrease. Centrifugal atomization uses a whirling disk to atomize the feed. The feed is ejected from the periphery of the disk at speeds ranging between 250 to 600 ft/sec (76.2 to 183 m/sec). Rotational speed of the wheel ranges from 3,000 to 20,000 rpm. Pressure atomization uses pressures between 100 to 7,000 psia (6.8 to 476 atm). Two fluid atomization uses air or steam at 60 to 100 psig (4 to 6.8 atm) to break up the feed into particles ranging from 10 to 20 microns in size. As in flash dryers, drying time is very short, from 3 to 10 seconds. This is due to the high degree of material dispersion in the gas stream which presents a maximum surface to it. Agitation is rapid, although not as much as in a flash dryer. Spray dryers have a distinct advantage over flash dryers, and fluidized-bed dryers in that spray dryers tend to shape the materials into spheroids. Advantages associated with spray dryers are: eliminates the need for intermediate steps such as filtering, crystallizing or centrifuging; shapes the dried product into spheroids of low bulk-density; minimum heat degradation due to short residence time; ability to process many different types of materials. Disadvantages associated with these dryers are: large space requirements; high initial capital cost; the low-bulk density of the product may be undesirable. Spray dryers have found acceptance in the chemical, pharmaceutical and food industries [60].

Direct Heat Drying Systems

In direct drying systems the product to be dried remains stationary in a bed or layer of material or is forced to fall through the heating medium. In the stationary bed mode, heat is transferred to the material by hot gases flowing across the bed. In this case moisture must diffuse to the top of the bed as the surface is dried by the air flowing across it. For the gases to flow through the bed, the particles being dried must agglomerate or be sufficiently permeable to allow passage of the gas. In the latter mode the material to be dried is gently tumbled by the rotation of the dryer, this facilitates the drying as the material remains loose. Drying rates are somewhat faster for this because a greater surface area is exposed to the heating medium. In general, direct heat dryers are suitable for operation with solids as most dryers in this category cannot handle liquids. For slurries, it is necessary to modify the dryer to accommodate recycling some of the processed material. There are three types of dryers in the direct heat systems. These are tunnel truck, turbotary, and rotary.

There are three types of tunnel dryers: tunnel truck dryers, belt conveyor dryer, vibrating conveyor dryers. The tunnel truck dryers employ trays in which to place the material to be dried. These are mounted one above the other on a truck. This arrangement permits easy loading and unloading of the trays and truck. This version of the tunnel dryer is used in the ceramic and porcelain enamel industries but finds little or no use in other indusries.

Belt conveyor dryers, vibrating and non-vibrating, operate by transporting the material to be dried across the dryer. This latter type of dryers lend themselves to continuous operation, however, maintenance requirements are somewhat higher than for tunnel dryers. Non-vibrating dryers are extensively used in the printing, textile and the flatwood stock industry. Vibrating dryers are mainly used in the food industry.

The turbo tray dryer is a continuous dryer made up of annular shelves stacked up one above the other. The drying is accomplished by vans rotating in the center section of the dryer which circulate air over the surface of the loaded trays into which each shelf is divided. The shelves also rotate and as the rotation proceeds, the wiper on each individual shelf pushes the material through radial slots onto the shelf below. The drying action on this dryer is similar to that of a tray dryer except that the material is periodically agitated. The agitation causes the wet material to be exposed continuously to the drying agent thus reducing the drying time considerably because the moisture does not have to diffuse through the full thickness of material on the tray. This type of dryer is utilized by the pharmaceutical, and the food and chemical processing industry. Advantages associated with this type of dryer are: its ability to handle materials from thick slurries (100,000 centipoise) to fine powders; space requirements are minimal; capable of split airstream to both dry and cool the stack; may be operated as a closed circuit system to recover vapors, or to dry in air inert atmosphere. Disadvantages associated with this type of dryer are: higher capital cost than in other types of dryers; prone to fouling of heating surfaces by dustry materials; dryer is unsuitable for materials that mat or for sticky substances.

A direct heat rotary dryer consists of a horizontal cylinder through which heated gas flows. The cylinder rotates and is generally inclined to the horizontal, so that the load can be made to flow by gravity. Usually the inside of the cylinder is equipped with flights running the entire length of the cylinder. These flights lift the material to be dried and shower it through the air stream. Ordinarily straight flights are used at the feed end of the dryer for sticky or wet materials. Forty-five degree and 90 degree flights are used with free flowing materials. Direct heat rotary dryers are used in the roasting of minerals, the chemical and the food industry. This type of dryer exhibits the following advantages: occluded moisture is readily removed because any reasonable retention time may be attained; reasonable capital cost; fairly close temperature control; drying and calcining may be carried out in the same unit; dryer may be operated with cocurrent or countercurrent flows. Disadvantages associated with this type of dryer are: large floor and building space requirements; requires dust collection units as very fine and dustry materials are blown out of the dryer [60].

Indirect Heat Dryers

Indirect heat dryers differ from direct heat dryers in that the heat transferred to the wet material is by conduction rather than convection or radiation. Indirect heat dryers are well suited for the recovery of solvents under reduced pressure and for avoiding explosive mixtures or oxidation of easily decomposed substances. Dusty materials are also handled easily. There are four types of dryers in the indirect heat systems. These are: rotary drum, vacuum, and vacuum freeze dryers.

Indirect heat rotary dryers work in much the same way as the direct heat rotary dryers. With one exception. In the indirect type, the heating medium and the material being processed are not allowed to come into contact with each other. Indirect-heat dryers are particularly useful in situations in which the material to be dried cannot be exposed to the combustion gases; or when sweeping the drying gases over the particulate material would cause excessive dusting; or when the liquid to be removed is a valuable solvent. Advantages associated with this type of dryer are: occluded moisture is readily removed; reasonable capital cost; fairly close temperature control. Disadvantages associated with this type of dryer are large space requirements.

Drum dryers consist of one or more horizontal rotating heated drums. The material to be dried is fed in amounts such that they form a thin layer that is scraped with adjustable blades, before one revolution is completed, off the surface of the drum. Drum dryers are classified as single, double, or twin drum units. The main difference between the double-drum dryer and the twin-drum is the direction of rotation. In the double drum dryer the tops of the drums rotate inwardly toward each other, whereas in the twin-drum type the rotation is away from each other. Drum dryers are particularly useful for processing materials which are too thick for spray dryers, and too thin for rotary dryers. Drum dryers are utilized in the chemical processing industry and in the food processing industry. A disadvantage of the double dryers is that it cannot process lumpy materials because these can be forced between the rolls with consequent damage to them, when this is the case twin drum dryers are used instead.

Vacuum dryers are utilized in the food and chemical industries for processing heat sensitive materials. Vacuum dryers rely on reduced operating pressures inside the drying chamber to effect the drying in a low temperature environment. These systems are particularly advantageous for: low temperature processing, solvent recovery, very low moisture content material, drying materials that combine with oxygen in the air. Disadvantages associated with these dryers are: high capital and maintenance costs and high operating cost [68,69].

Vacuum-freeze dryers are the most expensive and slowest of the drying processes, but they have some definite advantages over the other drying methods for many applications, especially in the food and pharmaceutical industries. These advantages are: little or no chemical change; loss of volatile components is minimized; the product dries without foaming; case hardening is eliminated; oxidation of the material is eliminated; sterility is maintained. Disadvantages associated with these dryers are: high capital cost, and high operating and maintenance cost [60].

Freeze Crystallization

Freeze separation processes are based on the difference in freezing point exhibited by the solvent and solute. As the solution is cooled, there is some temperature at which a solid crystalline begins to appear in the solution. Usually, only one component in the solution crystallizes, subsequently the volatile component (usually water) and the crystals are separated by other means. The crystals are then further purified. It is difficult to achieve high concentrations by freeze concentration. Liquid viscosity increases markedly as concentration increases and freezing point drops are so great that difficulty is experienced in handling the ice concentrate mixture and separating the concentrate from the ice. It is estimated that 35–50% dissolved solids represents the maximum concentration which can be reasonably obtained by freeze concentration. Freeze crystallization has not found widespread use in the industry due to high operating costs. Two developments in the area of crystallization, however, have contributed to make this technology a viable alternative to solvent recovery applications. First the use of direct contact evaporative refrigerants is overcoming heat transfer fouling, thus reducing investment in heat transfer surface and operating costs in cleaning. Second is the application of continuous countercurrent, solids washing column. Advantages associated with freeze drying are: low temperatures avoid chemical changes in unstable components; loss of volatile components is minimized; product may be dried without foaming; constituents of the dried material remain dispersed; coagulation of constituents is minimized; case-hardening is minimized; sterility is maintained; oxidation of the product is minimized or eliminated. Disadvantages associated with this technology are: not applicable to every separation problem; development work is needed on some of the simplified, less costly freeze cycles.

Fractional crystallization is a supersaturation phenomena achieved by cooling, partial evaporation of the solvent or addition of a precipitating agent. Seed crystals must be present (spontaneously or artificially induced) for crystallization to be initiated. Fractional crystallization is a series of crystallization usually in a column by the countercurrent contact between crystals and their melt. Crystals are melted and recrystallized a number of times yielding high quality crystals.

ELECTRIC METHODS

Electric technologies are rapidly replacing flame based processes in many industries. Besides its thermal capability, electricity as a motive force can be advantageously used in separating chemical species. Often electricity is used as an adjunct or an augmentation technique in fostering faster or more precise separations.

Electrophoresis

Differences in the mobility of ions and molecules in an electrical field can be exploited for separation. In a continuous flow zone electrophoresis, the mixture to be separated is continuously injected into a fluid between two electrodes. Individual species migrate sideways under the influence of the field creating zones that can be harvested downstream as separate fractions. A major problem (when using liquid rather than gel) is the presence of turbulence interfering with separation. In a new device, this problem is corrected by using a rotary system that stabilizes the flow of the carrier solution.

A single chambered continuous flow electrophoresis unit has flown on a shuttle flight. The zero gravity environment allowed a 500 times improved throughput while maintaining product purity.

New large scale electrophoresis apparatus have achieved purification of 40–50 grams of protein per hour or about 10^8 cells per minute. Power consumption is of the order of 3–6 kilowatt/hour. Such devices have not been tested for long term operation.

A modification to resolve ampholytes mixtures is based on differing isoelectric points rather than mobilities. When a pH gradient is established parallel to the field, each species migrate until it reaches the zone of its isoelectric point that is when it possesses no net surface charge. Isoelectric focusing is a technique allowing the separation of proteins differing but only slightly in their isoelectric points. It is sometimes used as a second step following polyacrylamide gel electrophoresis.

Electromagnetic Separation

Electromagnetic separation is based on the physical principle that unlike magnetic poles attract each other. When a particle is immersed in a magnetic field, a dipole field is induced in the particle and the field exerts a force on both ends of the particle. If the original field is constant, the forces on both ends of the particle will be equal but opposite and the particle will remain at rest. If the field has a gradient, then the force on one end of the particle will be larger than the force on the other end and the particle will be accelerated toward or away from the magnetic source depending on its magnetic properties. Ferromagnetic and paramagnetic materials are attracted and diamagnetic materials are repulsed. This principle can obviously be, and has been, used to separate magnetic from nonmagnetic materials. Recent advances have been in the perfection of apparatus that can deliver high magnetic fields and gradients so that even weakly magnetic materials may be separated; this has opened the door to a multitude of applications which could not be carried out with weak fields [19].

Electromagnetic separation may be used to separate magnetic as well as nonmagnetic particles. With magnetic particles, the process consists of passing the material near a divergent magnetic field, attracting the particles to the separator magnets and removing them. This has been effectively used in industry in: the removal of tramp iron from chemicals, food and lubricants; the beneficiation of iron ores to improve their grade; the beneficiation of other minerals; solid waste material recovery; the removal of magnetic materials from water effluents; coal desulfurization and ash removal.

With nonmagnetic particles, a magnetic seed is added together with a flocculant to the fluid to be treated. The flocculant binds the species to the magnetic seed particles forming flocs that can be separated using conventional electromagnetic separators. This method has been effectively used to remove suspended solids, bacteria, viruses and phosphates, and to modify the color and turbidity of river waters and discharges of sewage treatment plants. Results have been successful in demonstrating that magnetic separation in conjunction with other water treatment devices may be used to great advantage in water purification systems.

The separation of various blood components (red blood cells (RBC), platelets, etc.) is of considerable interest and use in specific therapeutic action and for research purposes. The removal of glycerol which is used in freezing to prevent crystallization is also of interest. The traditional tool for separation of blood components is the high-speed centrifuge. HGMS has been tested as an alternative. It is well established that oxyhaemoglobin is diamagnetic while deoxyhaemoglobin is paramagnetic. The magnetic susceptibility of crystalline ferrohaemoglobin has been estimated at 1.08×10^{-5} SI. The total susceptibility of totally reduced RBC has been estimated to be 3.88×10^{-6} assuming 3.4×10^{8} haemoglobin molecules/RBC. Using a laboratory device, the possibility of using HGMS to separate RBCs from other blood constituents was established. The low magnetic susceptibility of RBCs is offset by low flow rates. Under these conditions, plasma with low RBC or extremely pure red cells samples are obtained.

The manipulation of microcapsules (1–200 o.d.) containing enzymes or catalysts is described in two patent applications (3,954,666 and 3,954,678) by M. J. Marquisee and W. W. Prichard and assigned to Du Pont. The capsules are magnetic because of the incorporation of a ferromagnetic component allowing them to be manipulated by magnetic fields. The capsule walls are permeable, allowing the reactants and products to diffuse while retaining the catalyst or enzyme and the magnetic material.

Electrofiltration

This technique, applicable to dewatering fine particle material in a dilute dispersed environment, combines two well known technologies:

vacuum filtration and electrophoresis. In other words, the technique is essentially an electrically augmented vacuum filtration. In this process solids are electrodeposited on the anode in the form of a cake which is harvested from time to time. Filtrate is continuously removed from the cathode (which acts essentially as a filter) by the pressure differential.

Electrocoagulation

In many cases materials in solution is suspended by raising the pH and then precipitated. In contrast, if the solution is made on the acid side, the material coagulates and then is removed. Albumine can be made insoluble by coalescence. It has an isoelectric point, which can be reached by lowering the pH. When there is no more charge the albumine coalesces. Milk constituents can also be made insoluble and taken out this way. Usually pollutants are finely dispersed and carry a negative charge. To clear the effluent, one has to coagulate these particles, which is impossible unless one neutralizes their charge. Chemicals, such as aluminum and ferric sulfates, can be used for this purpose. Some industries, like the food industry, cannot utilize these chemicals when edible values are to be recovered either for human or for animal consumption. Electrocoagulation can achieve charge neutralization and achieve coagulation of suspended solids. At the same time, it gives buoyancy to the suspended and aggregated coagulates. This is due to:

a. High pH gradients at anode and cathode.
b. Evolution of gases, achieving uniform and controlled mixing action.
c. Transfer and neutralization of all electrostatic and ionic charges in the vicinity of the electrodes.

Electrostatic Separation

Electrostatic separation is used to separate granular solids having different electrical properties. The steps in electrostatic separation are essentially:

• charging of the feed particles
• exposing the charged particles to an electric field.

Three methods are available for charging powders made of dissimilar particles:

1. Rubbing—by vibrating or agitating the lot, results in paticles of one kind acquiring positive charges and the other kind negative ones. The metal plate against which the minerals rub must be grounded, to avoid creating a charge of opposite sign to the mineral which would

act as an electrostatic back pressure. If the plate is grounded, it can be used, in theory, to charge any quantity of material.

2. Spraying—Consists in passing the solid within a corona discharge between a wire (negatively charged) and an enclosure. The solids will be struck by the electrons and ions in the discharge and will emerge charged (Electrodynamic Separation).

3. Electrostatic Induction—on conducting particles situated on a grounded surface located in a high electrostatic potential. The conducting particles resting on the grounded surface will acquire charges on their side facing the high potential electrode, of sign contrary to the high potential, creating a lifting force.

Electrostatic separation devices are broadly of two kinds:

1. Free falling devices, where the particles fall vertically through a horizontal field maintained by two electrodes. Positively charged particles are deviated towards the cathode, negative ones towards the anode. This device is best suited for particles charged by mutual friction. Some devices are of an off-center pattern, permitting particles to strike a conducting wall, whereby separation is between conductors and non-conductors rather than positively and negatively charged particles.

2. Drum devices, consisting of two drums, one of larger diameter, which brings the feed into the electric field, and the other of lesser diameter, which provides the high potential electrode. In addition, modern devices have a corona electrode to spray the solid particles with ions. Separation is primarily between conductors and non-conductors.

As separation depends on the charge acquired by particle surface it strongly depends on particle size. The particle surface varies as the square of radius, the volume (and weight) as the cube. The competition between weight and charge favors small particles. The size range of the feed may have to be narrow if the two powders have close electrical properties. A broader spectrum of particle size may be separated if the powders have dissimilar electric properties.

Electromagnetic Energy Dryers

Included in this category are infrared (IR) dryers, and microwave (MW) dryers. IR dryers operate by heating the surface of the material to be dried. IR dryers are suitable for drying even, flat surfaces. On bulky materials where the surface tends to be broken and rough, the unevenness causes the drying to be non-uniform. MW systems take advantage of the fact that water molecules are excited by electromagnetic waves of certain wavelength. MW systems are impervious to the class of material to be dried.

CONCLUSION

In a typical industrial environment, the reactant and the product as well as by-products and impurities are in the same phase. This phase is usually a gas on a liquid. The product is often very diluted. This high dilution and easy cohabitation are a challenge to the scientist and technician.

Much effort goes into developing separation, purification and concentration unit operations based on the physical-chemical properties of the molecules in a mixture (volatility, adsorption, solubility, etc.).

Recovery costs of products are important. They are twice the cost of fermentation for enzyme products, the same for penicillin and one-sixth for ethanol.

Most separation techniques must deal with very dilute solution. Dewatering becomes an important step to limit the volume that must be handled by more costly and time consuming methods.

Chemical engineers are attempting to duplicate on a large scale what chemists can produce in small quantities. Large scale industrial processes are often very dissimilar from those used in small scale laboratory production. Dominant economic factors and technical scale-up difficulties are the turning points.

In biotechnology like in other application areas and in separation, like in any other industrial operation, the trend is to do it cheaper, faster, make it more selective and sensitive, combine it with other methods, miniaturize it and automate it. These trends are intensifying as new applications deal with larger, more complex and fragile molecules to be isolated from a complex mixture.

Separation cannot be an afterthought and must be integrated in the design. Since both fermentation and separation are affected differently by the same parameters, a compromise solution must be sought [70].

The temperature and pH of the broth, the presence of antifoaming and precipitation agents, the ionic strength of the solution, the presence of remaining raw material at the harvesting time, the distribution of the desired products (intracellular vs. extracellular), the viscosity of the broth and the nature of interfering solids must all be taken into account.

The situation is made more complex by a normally very dilute solution and the presence of very similar chemical species (in terms of structure, reactivity and properties). The problem is compounded by increasing demand for higher purity and activity of the isolated product, the tendency for larger scaled-up operation, and the rising role of energy, raw material and equipment in the overall cost [21].

Several methods will be used in series and parallel in an integrated separation system for instance ultrafiltration, electrophoresis and reverse osmosis can be effectively combined in alcohol production process for preconcentration, desalting, alcohol removal, yeast cell concentration, etc.

A few predictions are made for the near future:

- Ion exchange (IE) will probably remain the most prevalent practice in the U.S. for some time to come. IE columns are simple to operate and most plants already have IE capacity.
- Thermal methods will require some form of energy recovery in order to remain competitive.
- Electrotechnologies, because of their ease of automation and capability for fine control, will make rapid gains.
- Supercritical fluid extraction, once demonstrated on a commercial scale, should take its place among valuable separation techniques.
- Membrane methods will gain wide access and be applied to an expanding realm of problems.
- The transition from the laboratory, to the pilot plant, to the commercial facility will not be easy but is required for many existing sensitive techniques.
- Automation and process control will become the norm rather than the exception.
- Engineering intensification know how for higher efficiency, greater throughput, lower cost, reduced energy needs, will be systematically applied to existing and evolving techniques.
- More synergism between separate fields and more work at the interface between technical disciplines will take place.
- New electric preparative methods will invade the market. Within the last five years, techniques such as force flow electrophoresis (electrophoresis conducted through a membrane as opposed to the conventional method, i.e., through an agar gel) and isoelectric focus (preparative technique not more than two years old involving movement across a pH gradient with well defined isoelectric points) have been developed as preparative methods derived from the analytical field. Free-flow electrophoresis (movement of cells through an electrical field, not a membrane) developed at the Max Planck Institute is being used at investigative clinics throughout the U.S. The future of isoelec-

tric focusing free and force flow electrophoresis is probably dependent on the need for the drugs produced which will be administered in nanogram quantities and are expensive to produce. These processes, do, however, provide a much more precise separation (200–400 molecular weight) than does ultrafiltration (200–300 molecular weight).

• Affinity methods are likely to play a more important role in the future because of the possibility to raise antibodies against virtually any protein of interest.

If a conclusion can be drawn from this survey, it is that a vast arsenal of proven techniques are available. Biotechnology will create a high demand for such techniques and will foster the development of new ones to the benefit of all industries.

REFERENCES

1. Porter, M. C., "A Novel Membrane Filter for the Laboratory," *American Laboratory* (November 1974).

2. Sassaman, J. F., "Membrane Technology in Industry," WP82W00223 (April 1982).

3. Baum, B., W. Holley, Jr., and R. A. White, "Hollow Fibres in Reverse Osmosis, Dialysis, and Ultrafiltration," in *Membrane Separation Processes*, P. Meareas, ed., pp. 187–229, Elsevier Scientific Publishing Company, New York (1976).

4. Sammon, D. C., "The Treatment of Aqueous Wastes and Foods by Membrane Processes," in *Membrane Separation Processes*, P. Meares, ed., pp. 499–528, Elsevier Scientific Publishing Company, New York (1976).

5. *Chemical Engineering*, 19 (August 22, 1983).

6. Harris, F. L., G. B. Humphreys, and K. S. Spiegler, "Reverse Osmosis (Hyperfiltration) in Water Desalination," in *Membrane Separation Processes*, P. Meares, ed., pp. 121–186, Elsevier Scientific Publishing Company, New York (1976).

7. Lee, T. S., D. Omstead, N.-H. Lu, and H. R. Gregor, "Membrane Separations in Alcohol Production," *Ann. NY Acad. Sci., 369*, 367–381 (1981).

8. Howell, J. A., O. Velicangil, M. S. Le, and A. L. Herrera Zeppelin, "Ultrafiltration of Protein Solutions," *Ann. NY Acad. Sci., 369*, 355–366 (1981).

9. Porter, M. C. and J. H. Schneider, "Nucleopore Membranes for Air and Liquid Filtration," *Filtration Engineering* (January/February 1973).

10. Spurny, K. R., J. P. Lodge, Jr., E. R. Frank, and D. C. Sheesley, "Aerosol Filtration by Means of Nucleopore Filters—Structural and Filtration Properties," *Environmental Science and Technology, 3* (5), 453–464 (1969).

11. Li, N. N., U.S. Patent 3,410,794, issued 12 November 1968.

12. Joglekar, R., "Survey of Liquid Membranes and Membrane Alternatives to Distillation," WP82W0233 (April 1982).

13. Cahn, R. D. and N. N. Li, "Separation of Phenol from Waste Water by the Liquid Membrane Technique," *Separation Science, 9* (6), 505–519 (1974).

14. Stannett, V. T., W. J. Koros, D. R. Paul, M. K. Lonsdale, and R. W. Baker, "Recent Advances in Membrane Science and Technology," *Advances in Polymer Science, 32,* 69–121 (1979).

15. Herbert, W. J., British Patent No. 1,080,994 (1967).

16. Davis, S. S., "Liquid Membranes and Multiple Emissions," *Chemistry and Industry,* 683–687 (3 October 1981).

17. Zhu, C. L., C. W. Yuang, J. R. Fried, and D. B. Greenberg, "Pervaporization Membranes—A Novel Separation Technique for Trace Organics," *Environmental Progress, 2* (2), 132–143 (1983).

18. Stern, S. A., "The Separation of Gases by Selective Permeation," in *Membrane Separation Processes,* P. Meares, ed., pp. 295–326, Elsevier Scientific Publishing Company, New York (1976).

19. Ouellette, R. P., J. A. King, and P. N. Cheremisinoff, *Electrotechnology, Vol. 1,* Wastewater Treatment and Separation Methods, Ann Arbor Science Publishers, Inc. (1978).

20. Larson, A., "Various Approaches to the Separation Process for Harvesting the Products of Fermentation in the Field of Antibiotics in Advances in Microbial Engineering," *Biotechnology and Bioengineering Symposium, 4,* 917–931 (1974).

21. Jefferis, R. P., III, "Control of Biochemical Recovery Processes," *Ann. NY Acad. Sci., 369,* 275–284 (1981).

22. Round, J. J., R. B. Liptak, and W. C. McGregor, "Continuous-Flow Ultracentrifugation in Preparative Biochemistry," *Ann. NY Acad. Sci., 369,* 265–274 (1981).

23. Griffith, W. L., A. L. Compere, C. G. Westmoreland, and J. S. Johnson, "Separation of Biopolymer from Fermentation Broths," in *Synthetic Membranes: Vol. II,* A. F. Turbak, ed., ACS Symposium Series 1959, American Chemical Society, Washington, D.C. (1981).

24. Garg, D. R. and J. P. Ausikaitis, "Molecular Sieve Dehydration Cycle for High Water Content Streams," *CEP,* 60–65 (April 1983).

25. Orichowsky, S. T., C. R. Wilke, and H. W. Blanch, "Recovery of Cellulase Enzymes by Countercurrent Adsorption," Dept. of Chemical Engineering and Lawrence Berkeley Laboratory, University of California, Berkeley, CA 94720, LBL-15153 (1982).

26. Hone, R. W., M. Lamerchand, and W. Malaty, "Separation of Water-Ethanol Mixtures by Sorption, Part 2," ORNL/MIT-304, Oak Ridge National Laboratory, Oak Ridge, Tenn. (1981).

27. Schneider, M., C. Guillot, and B. Lamy, "The Affinity Precipitation Technique. Application to the Isolation and Purification of Trypsin from Bovine Pancreas," *Ann. NY Acad. Sci., 369,* 257–263 (1981).

28. Kula, M.-R., K. H. Kroner, H. Hustedt, and H. Schutte, "Technical Assets of Extractive Enzyme Purification," *Ann. NY Acad. Sci., 369,* 341–354 (1981).

29. Sood, S., "Application of Supercritical CO_2," WP81W00121, The MITRE Corp. (January 1982).

30. "System is Designed for Critical-Fluid Extractions," *Chemical Engineering,* 33 (January 25, 1982).

31. Sims, M., "Process Uses Liquid CO_2 for Botanical Extractions," *Chemical Engineering,* 50–51 (January 25, 1982).

32. Caragay, A. B. and V. Krukonis, "Supercritical Fluid Extraction for Purification and Fractionation of Fats and Oils," Paper presented at the 72nd Annual Meeting of American Oil Chemists Society, New Orleans, LA (18 May 1981).

33. Hubert, P. and O. G. Vitzhum, "Fluid Extraction of Hops, Spices and Tobacco with Supercritial Gasers," in *Extraction with Supercritical Gases,* G. M. Schneider, E. Stahl, and G. Wilke, eds., pp. 25–43, Verlag Chemie, Weinheim, West Germany (1980).

34. Hag, A. G., "Method for Producing Hop Extracts," British Patent, 1,388,581 (1971).

35. Zosel, K., "Separation with Supercritical Gases: Practical Applications," in *Extraction with Supercritical Gases,* G. M. Schneider, E. Stahl, and G. Wilkes, eds., pp. 1–23, Verlag Chemie, Weinheim, West Germany (1980).

36. Worthy, W., "Gases at High Pressure and Above Critical Temperature Separate Compounds Under Mild Conditions, Require Less Energy but More Capital," *Chemical and Engineering News,* 16–17 (3 Aug., 1981).

37. "Gas Solvents: About to Blast Off," *Business Week,* 68M (27 July 1981).

38. Mowery, R. A., E. N. Fuller, and R. K. Bade, "On-Line Process Size-Exclusion Chromatography," *American Laboratory,* 61–67 (May 1982).

39. Hearn, T. W., T. E. Regnier, and C. T. Wehr, "HALC of Peptides and Proteins," *American Laboratory,* 18–39 (October 1982).

40. Raja, R., "Metal Ion Liquid Chromatography," *American Laboratory,* 35–37 (July 1982).

41. Zief, M., L. J. Crane, and J. Horvath, "Preparation of Steroid Samples by Solid-Phase Extraction," *American Laboratory,* 120–130 (May 1982).

42. Zief, M., L. J. Crane, and J. Horvath, "Low-Pressure Preparative Liquid Chromatography," *American Laboratory,* 144–153 (March 1982).

43. Richey, J., "FPLC: A Comprehensive Separation Technique for Biopolymers," *American Laboratory,* 104–129 (October 1982).

44. *Chemical Engineering,* 18 (August 22, 1983).

45. DiCesare, J. L., "Control of Column Properties Makes LC Fast and Efficient," *Ind. Res. & Develop.,* 130–133 (March 1983).

46. DiCesare, J. L. and F. L. Vandemark, "Automated HPLC Separates Samples in Lab Quantities," *Ind. Res. & Develop.,* 138–141 (Feb. 1982).

47. Lehrer, R., "Hall's Artificial Intelligence Gives Quality Separation," *Ind. Res. & Develop.,* 116–119 (April 1969).

48. Gudkin, M. and V. Patel, "Aqueous Gel Filtration Chromatography of Enzymes, Proteins, Oligosaccharides, and Nucleic Acids," *American Laboratory,* 64–73 (January 1982).

49. Mandava, N. B., Y. Ito, and W. D. Conway, "Countercurrent Chromatography I: Historical Development and Early Instrumentation," *American Laboratory,* 62–78 (October 1982).

50. Mandava, N. B., Y. Ito, and W. D. Conway, "Countercurrent Chromatography II: Recent Instrumentation and Applications," *American Laboratory,* 48–57 (1982).

51. Dunnill, P. and M. D. Lilly, "Recent Developments in Enzyme Isolation Process," *Enzyme Engineering, Vol. 2,* E. K. Pye and L. B. Wingard, eds., Plenum Press (1975).

52. Anderson N. G., D. W. Holladay, J. E. Caton, and J. W. Holleman, "Protein

Purification by Immunoadsorption," in *Enzyme Engineering, Vol. 2,* E. K. Pye and L. B. Wingard, eds., Plenum Press (1975).

53. Pestka, S., "The Purification and Manufacture of Human Interferons," *Sci. Amer., 249* (2), 37–43 (1983).

54. Bonnafous, J.-C., J. Dornand, J. Favero, M. Sizes, E. Boschetti, and J.-C. Mani, "Cell Affinity Chromatography with Ligands Immobilized Through Cleavable Mercury-Sulfur Bonds," *J. Immunological Methods, 58,* 93–107 (1983).

55. Basch, R. S., J. W. Berman, and E. Lakow, "Cell Separation Using Positive Immunoselective Techniques," *J. Immunological Methods, 56,* 269–280 (1983).

56. Mix, T. J., T. S. Dweek, and M. Weinberg, "Energy Conservation in Distillation," *Chemical Engineering Progress, 74* (4), 49–55 (1978).

57. Kenney, W. F., "Reducing the Energy Demand of Separation Processes," *Chemical Engineering Progress, 75* (3), 68–71 (1979).

58. Joglekar, R., "Survey of Vapor Recompression Applications in Industry," WP82W00234, The MITRE Corp. (June 1982).

59. *Chemical Engineering News,* 15 (July 11, 1983).

60. Muradaz, M., "State of the Art of Industrial Drying," WP80W00742, The MITRE Corp. (February 1981).

61. Dinnage, D. F., "How to Design for Economic Evaporation," *Ford Engineering, 47* (12), 51–54 (1975).

62. Rosenblad, A. E., Personal communication. A memo: Chemical Processing Inquiry and Product Brochure dated May. Rosenblad Corporation, Princeton, NJ (1981).

63. Rozycki, J., "Energy Conservation via Recompression Evaporation," *Chemical Engineering Progress, 72* (5), 69–72 (1976).

64. Cole, J. W., "Mechanical Vapor Recompression for Evaporators," *Chemical Engineering,* 76–78 and 81 (February 1975).

65. Root, W. L., III, "Indirect Drying of Solids," *Chemical Engineering,* 52–64 (May 2, 1983).

66. Beddow, J. K., "Dry Separation Techniques," *Chemical Engineering,* 70–84 (August 10, 1981).

67. Mortensen, S. and S. Hovmand, "Fluidized-Bed Spray Granulation," *CEP,* 37–42 (April 1983).

68. Freeman, M. P., "Vacuum Electrofiltration," *CEP,* 74–79 (August 1982).

69. Forthuber, D., "Continuous Vacuum Plate Dryer," *CEP,* 71–76 (April 1983).

70. Paul, E. L., A. Kaufman, and W. A. Sklarz, "An Industrial Approach to Integrated Fermentation Isolation Process Development," *Ann. NY Acad. Sci., 367,* 181–186 (1981).

12

Computers and Biotechnology

INTRODUCTION

ife is probably the most complex of processes; hence a new family of computerized instruments is needed to analyze and understand its manifestations. Molecular biology has a language, a grammar, a logic, and a mathematics of its own, and biological and computer languages have much in common. Biotechnology is a way of dealing with large numbers related to cells, amino acids, nucleotide bases, and molecules. Biotechnololgy is not only a science, but also a business; therefore it must scale-up its production facilities and control the quality of its products.

For all these reasons and more, the marriage between biotechnology and computer science is a fortuitous one, likely to stimulate, nurture, and expand both areas of human knowledge. Without computers, biotechnology would be progressing slowly and painfully, rather than exploding as it is today.

DATA BASES

Most technical papers in molecular biology present DNA/RNA sequences. The reader is subjected, line after line, to A,T,C,G's. The utility of such papers is doubtful, and there are many difficulties in manipulating the information and avoiding errors in transcription.

It is not surprising that there have been many attempts to record these findings in computer-based systems. More than 500,000 bases covering the entire living kingdom have been reported in the scientific literature;

about 1,000 proteins have been characterized in some detail. Since the advent of the Maxam/Gilbert and Sanger methods, it has become relatively easy to sequence a length of DNA or RNA in minimum time and with great accuracy.

A few organisms genomes have been totally sequenced. These include the bacteriophage fd (6,408 bases); the coliovirus (7,433 bases); the cauliflower mosaic virus (8,024 bases); the Moloney murine leukemia virus (18,332); ϕX124 (5,386 bases); SV40 (5,226 bases); the Rous Sarcoma virus (9,302 bases). The longest sequence known is 16,569 bases, for the human mitochondrion (SGC1) genome. If one considers that a human cell probably contains some 50,000 different proteins, it is clear that much more is to come. The well-known E. coli bacteria is estimated to contain 5 million bases in its genome; while this is certainly a challenge, each of the 46 chromosomes of the human cell is estimated to contain about 500 million bases.

The Department of Health and Human Services is sponsoring design and deployment of a national data bank for DNA sequences, with the actual design work contracted to Bolt Beranek and Newman. The most important data banks in operation are shown in Table 12-1.

The existence of these large-scale data banks of crystallographic data, protein sequences, and nucleic acid sequences does not preclude the existence of specialized smaller libraries. Examples of the latter are the

TABLE 12-1. Data Bases.

Data Bank	Organization	Status	Availability Mag Tape	On-line
	National Biomedical Research Found. Washington, D.C.	557,000 nucleotides 500 sequences	X	X
Nucleotide Sequence Data Lib.	European Molecular Biology Lab (EML) Heidelberg, FRG	600,000 nucleotides 600 sequences	X	X
Two-dimens. Gel maps	Argonne Natl. Lab Argonne, IL			
Brookhaven Protein Data Bank	Brookhaven Natl. Lab	47 Macromolecules	X	
	Cambridge Crystallographic Data Ctr.			
Los Alamos Sequence Lib.	Los Alamos Natl. Lab, University of Cal.	486,000 nucleotides 320 sequences		X

library at the University of Colorado (DELILA System), a specialized tRNA data base at Wichita State University, and a comprehensive compilation of tRNA sequences at the Max Planck Institute for Experimental Medicine.

RESTRICTION ENZYMES

Endonucleases are an essential part of the mechanism that protects bacterial cells from viral attack; they do this by degrading foreign DNA. Several hundreds of these enzymes are known and commercially available. The Type II ones are especially interesting since their recognition site is four to six nucleotide long and they have two-fold positional symmetry (diad symmetry). These enzymes can digest DNA sequences in a variety of lengths.

Restriction enzymes are essential to genetic engineering since they are at the heart of gene manipulation. The cutting enzymes are also a powerful analytical tool in sequencing DNA; they have been used to compare DNA sequences from related organisms and to infer phylogenetic relationships. A number of statistical methods and computer programs have been developed to enhance their usefulness. Current efforts are concentrated on developing strategies for minimizing the number of gel runs and sequencing reactions. The ordering of restriction fragments and the mapping of the sites on a circular or linear map are well established.

GEL SEQUENCING

Available DNA sequencing methods permit the resolution of products up to chain lengths of 250 to 300 nucleotides on thin polyacrylamide gels. The four channels of the autoradiograph can be read easily, permitting reconstruction of the original sequence. The tedious and time-consuming nature of this operation, together with the substantial probability of error associated with any manual method of recording information, has led scientists to develop automated techniques. Using a digitizing tablet, it is possible to record automatically the location of any point on a gel, thus avoiding most of these problems. At least two such systems are in use: in the Cold Spring Harbor Laboratory's DIGI-PAD system, a translucent digitizing tablet is connected to a PDP 11/44 minicomputer; at the National Cancer Institute, a graphic tablet is connected to a Tectronic 4002 computer.

One way to approach the DNA sequencing of large molecules is to sequence unmapped fragments derived from restriction enzyme digestion. If the total DNA sequence is to be generated from this fragmentary information, subtle analysis is required. A number of computer programs perform this feat, working interactively with the scientist in the laboratory.

SEQUENCE ANALYSIS

Once DNA sequences are available in computer form, they can undergo various kinds of mathematical and statistical manipulation and analysis. Computer programs are available to perform the following functions:

- Generate lists of restriction sites and construct restriction maps.
- Translate the DNA code into amino acid sequences, in the three possible reading frames.
- Discover homologic relations between sequences.
- Perform a variety of statistical analyses, including codon usage (distribution of triplets) and amino acid distribution.
- Display this information in tabular and graphical forms.

The most valuable application of these pattern recognition programs is in the analysis of newly discovered sequence of unknown functions. The first task is to identify the initiation and termination codon and the proper reading frame. The next task is to separate coding from noncoding regions. Fickett, Rodier, Shepherd, and others have developed codes to perform such analyses with greater speed and accuracy. Through the use of such techniques, the role and function of the vast amount of noncoding DNA should be elucidated shortly.

Using such methods, intron/exon boundaries have been characterized; the components of operons (e.g., promotor, repressor), have been defined; and ribosome binding sites have been identified. Symmetric patterns (palindromic regions, inverted repeats) are rapidly identified; the fact that they occur more frequently than is predicted by random theory indicates control regions in the sequence. Correlation methods have revealed beautiful cycles and periodicities in sequences, some clearly associated with the physics of the twisted double helix, others of unknown origin.

MOLECULAR BIOLOGY LANGUAGES

Molecular biology has evolved rapidly in recent years. Likewise, there has been a proliferation of computer programs, including applications, algorithms, languages, and host computers. With this diversity, the biologist must become a computer specialist to make full use of the available capabilities. Consequently, a molecular biology computer language for the naive computer user is needed. A number of such efforts are underway. Most notable are the DNA language of the University of Wisconsin, and the GENESIS system, which is part of the MOLGEN project at Stanford University. These languages and their expected progeny will make extensive use of recent findings in artificial intelligence and knowledge based systems.

Many commercial firms have dedicated themselves to developing and distributing computer software of interest to molecular biologists and biotechnologists. Among these efforts, EAN-TECH and Intelligenetics are the most prominent.

RNA'S SECONDARY STRUCTURE

A number of computer programs have been developed to compute and display the secondary structures of mRNA and tRNA based on primary sequences. Most predictive models in use today employ a thermodynamic energy minimization algorithm. A series of thermodynamic studies has defined the free energy of stacked base pairs and single stranded regions in hairpin loops, bulges, and internal loops. The rules for energy minimization have been codified by I. Tinoco Jr.

THE STRUCTURE OF PROTEINS

Proteins are sequences of amino acids. It is commonplace to define their level of organization as primary, secondary, tertiary, and quartery structures:

• The primary structure is the actual sequence of amino acids.
• The formation of secondary structures relies on hydrogen bonding.
• Helical structures and parallel and anti-parallel sheet structures are almost universally present in proteins; tertiary structures result from

the packing or assembly of helices and sheets. The protein is normally biologically active only when folded in its tertiary form.

• The quartery structure is the organization of the protein into well-defined domains.

A vast literature exists on modeling and predicting the secondary and tertiary structures of proteins.

The prediction of secondary structures has reached an accuracy of some 60%. An accuracy of about 70% is achieved if the recognition of super secondary structures is incorporated, which appears to be the state of the art. Most of this work can be traced to the seminal efforts of Chou and Fasman, which provided probabilities for helices and sheets for the 20 amino acid residues.

The problem of identifying the self assembly of secondary structures into a tertiary structure is compounded by a lack of definitive and visible criteria. A number of rules have been applied, with some success.

• Proteins contain a hydrophobic core (Kauzmann).
• The native structure of a protein is a configuration of minimum free energy.
• The residues buried in the interior of a protein are tightly packed.
• Folding occurs along closely defined pathways during synthesis.
• Specific structures are present (e.g., hydrophobic regions, disulfide bridges, etc.).

Using x-ray diffraction techniques, the tertiary structure of about 100 proteins has been determined. Two basic methods are generally used to predict tertiary structure.

• Based on a high level of detail (the location of various atoms of the molecule), an energy minimization function is reached by brute force. This function is nonlinear and contains a large number of terms. Contact maps, and generally distance maps, are computed based on short- and long-range interactions.
• Using a low level of details and a simplified energy function, a gross approximation of the structure is obtained; this is refined with additional information.

ENZYME ACTIVITY MODELING

Computer modeling is being applied extensively to such problems of chemistry and biochemistry as the following: chemical kinetics, membrane transport phenomena, drug-receptor dynamics, structure-activity relationships, drug design, antigen-antibody interaction, and bio-molecular sub-assembly. The ultimate goal is to understand the activity of proteins and direct them against substrates of interest. A number of experimental studies on structure activity relationships have provided much empirical evidence on the location of the active site and the basis for catalysis. *Ab initio* molecular orbital calculations have been completed for the active sites of some enzymes, providing insight into the field effects on molecular catalysis.

Protein scientists have for years built "stick-and-ball" models of proteins to obtain a visual, three-dimensional representation of large molecules. However, the advent of computers with sophisticated, multicolor graphics terminals and software has made possible the display and manipulation of large molecules with minimum effort; enzyme-substrate interactions can also be shown. The most sophisticated systems give the image a three-dimensional impression by projecting of coordinates onto a matrix; the use of intensity control also enhances the depth effect.

Although static pictures are very useful, the dynamics of interaction are what interests us the most. The capability of the computer to change atomic distances and bond angles through rotation allows us to bring the molecules to life. By concentrating on features of interest, such as an active site, and combining color and movement, we can achieve the greatest insight into protein behavior, activity, and interactions. Color terminals are available from numerous firms, including Tektronix, Hewlett-Packard, Calcomp, Zeta, Servogor, Ramtek, ADI, IBM, and Chromatics. Software graphics packages are available with all color terminals, as is such general-purpose software as SAS/GRAPH.

PHYLOGENETIC TREES

One of the goals of biology is to reconstruct the past events that gave rise to the diversity of proteins now in existence. It is assumed that most enzymes evolved from a small set of archetypal proteins through duplications and modifications. The development of a phylogenetic tree from a data set is a problem of graph theory. The evolutionary relation (in the form of a distance) among a set of proteins is of much interest in the reconstruction of the presumed evolutionary path. The construction of such trees permits the statistical testing of competing evolution theories.

The exploration of sequence relationships involves three steps. First, a data base of protein sequences for many species must be available. The optimum alignment of amino acid sequences involves a gap penalty each time a skip is made in one or another protein to ensure alignment. Second, a numerical score must be computed, often in the form of a distance measure. This distance measure, or similarity index, is often derived in terms of minimum mutation rates. Finally, starting with the distance measure in the form of a matrix, an approximate tree is produced and refined by successive pairwise clustering. Without the use of computers, such manipulation of large data sets and the production of dendritic trees would be impossible, except for small and trivial cases. A variety of computer programs are available for computing distance matrices and displaying evolutionary trees.

AUTOMATION

Digital computers were first used for close loop control in aircraft flight control in 1955; for monitoring in an electric utility in 1958; for supervisory control in a refinery in 1959; and for operations in a chemical plant in 1960. The total of digital computers installed in industrial control applications since the 1960s is more than 500,000 units, with an annual growth rate of over 65%. Some 250,000 new units will be added this year, and control applications will account for 20% of all computer uses.

The most significant trend in computer technology over the last 25 years has been the reduced size of the computer. Machines have shrunk from mainframe to minicomputer to microcomputer, to a single circuit chip with complete logical processing and memory capability. There have been correspondingly dramatic decreases in the price of having a computer perform a given function or operation: the cost of computers dropped three to four orders of magnitude from the early 1960s to the present. Other improvements have combined to make automation an attractive possibility, and often a necessity. Computer reliability has increased to the point of less than one system component failure per year. Memory has expanded in size and speed of access. Equipment has been transformed from basically analog to basically digital throughout the industry to adapt to the digital computer.

Other developments have made computers easier to use. Systems now commonly operate in real time rather than in a batch mode. Compiler languages have become easier to master, and programming languages are user-friendly. Interactive capability through a console provides rapid access to the central computing power and data bases at remote locations. On the other hand, the availability of personnel trained to use and program the computer remains a problem. Moreover, hardware has outpaced software, and software is often not utilized optimally by the user.

The parameters most often measured in an industrial environment are temperature and pressure. Timing, counting, force, torque, acceleration, position, pH, moisture, density, and chemical composition are often measured in process control applications. Most analytical instruments available in the laboratory and in the process industry provide digital output, and more than one sophisticated device has its own minicomputer on-board. Process control valves, electric motors and drives, hydraulic servos, and fluid power are the most frequently used actuation devices.

Computers are employed to perform four functions: process monitoring, analysis, control, and optimization. In the field of biotechnology, we are interested in measuring and controlling pH, temperature, dissolved oxygen, redox potential, substrate concentrations, product concentrations, mass flow rate, heat evolution, gaseous oxygen and carbon dioxide concentrations, cell mass, enzyme levels, and cofactors (ATP, NAD/NADH) activity. As of now, computers are used mostly to monitor and control the fermentation step. A not-so-high level of sophistication has been achieved in dealing with the single, independent, closed-loop feedback control of culture conditions such as temperature, pH, and dissolved oxygen. The reason for this state of affairs is the difficulty of applying sensors developed in other fields, as well as the challenges associated with data interpretation. Few of the sensors available can directly measure biological properties at the plant-scale level in a heterogeneous environment.

The development of biological electrodes, ions, and chemical field effect transistors will do much to improve this situation. These devices can be made specific, sensitive, rugged, small, rapid, and inexpensive. Ultimately, we may expect to see the simultaneous monitoring and control of multiple parameters, simulation, and process modeling, as well as real optimization based upon reference models. Such capabilities have been achieved in other, more mature, fields.

Automation in biotechnology will continue to be influenced by the general trend in the computer industry toward smaller, less expensive systems, greater ease of interaction between computer and operator, and reduced computer-system-caused downtime. In monitoring devices, the trend is toward faster and more accurate sensors, particularly of the electronic type.

CONCLUSIONS

Computers and biotechnology are the two phenomena likely to have the largest impact on people living in this century. It is not surprising that their relationship is synergistic, and that the product of their joint effort is a challenge to many minds. Future generations of scientists will fail to understand how the biotechnologists of today achieved such success with such primitive tools. With limited imagination, we can predict computers involved in designing experiments, developing strategies and testing schemes, analyzing results, and projecting new options and possibilities. On a more mundane level, much of the routine work of biotechnology (sequencing, pattern recognition, information storage, monitoring of experiments) will be left to the computer, freeing the technologist to go back to nature and the laboratory where his work began.

REFERENCES

1. Aaronson, R. P., J. F. Young, and P. Palese, "Oligonucleotide Mapping: Evaluation of Its Sensitivity by Computer-Simulation," *Nucleic Acids Research, 10* (1), 237-246 (1982).

2. Auron, P. E., W. P. Rindone, C. P. H. Vary, J. J. Celentano, and J. N. Vournakis, "Computer-Aided Prediction of RNA Secondary Structures," *Nucleic Acids Research, 10* (1), 403-419 (1982).

3. Azbel, M. Y., Y. Kantor, L. Verkh, and A. Vilenkin, "Statistical Analysis of DMA Sequencies. I.," *Biopolymers, 21,* 1687-1690 (1982).

4. Bach, R., P. Friedland, D. L. Brutlag, and L. Kedes, "MAXAMIZE. A DNA Sequencing Strategy Advisor," *Nucleic Acids Research, 10* (1), 295-304 (1982).

5. Bello, J., "Stability of Protein Conformation: Internal Packing and Enthalpy of Fusion of Model Compounds," *J. Theor. Biol., 68,* 139-142 (1977).

6. Blumenthal, R. M., P. J. Rice, and R. J. Roberts, "Computer Programs for Nucleic Acid Sequence Manipulation," *Nucleic Acids Research, 10* (1), 91-101 (1982).

7. Brutlag, D. L., J. Clayton, P. Friedland, and L. H. Kedes, "SEQ: A Nucleotide Sequence Analysis and Recombination System," *Nucleic Acids Research, 10* (1), 279-294 (1982).

8. Brandts, J. F., M. Brennan, and L. N. Lin, "Unfolding and Refolding Occur Much Faster for a Proline-Free Protein Than for Most Proline-Containing Proteins," *Proc. Natl. Acad. Sci., 74* (10), 4178-4181 (1977).

9. Charton, M., "Protein Folding and the Genetic Code: An Alternative Quantitative Model," *J. Theor. Biol., 91,* 115-123 (1981).

10. Chothia, C., M. Levitt, and D. Richardson, "Structure of Proteins: Packing of A-Helices and Pleated Sheets," *Proc. Natl. Acad. Sci., 74* (10), 4130-4134 (1977).

11. Chou, P. Y. and G. D. Fasman, "Prediction of Protein Conformation," *Biochemistry, 13* (2), 222-244 (1974).

12. Clayton, J. and L. Kedes, "GEL, A DNA Sequencing Project Management System," *Nucleic Acids Research, 10* (1), 305-321 (1982).

13. Connolly, M. L., "Solvent-Accessible Surfaces of Proteins and Nucleic Acids," *Science, 221* (4612), 709-713 (1983).

14. Conrad, B. and D. W. Mount, "Microcomputer Programs for DNA Sequence Analysis," *Nucleic Acids Research, 10* (1), 31-38 (1982).

15. Corrigan, A. J. and P. C. Huang, "A BASIC Microcomputer Program for Plotting the Secondary Structure of Proteins," *Computer Programs in Biomedicine, 15,* 163-168 (1982).

16. Delaney, A. D., "A DNA Sequence Handling Program," *Nucleic Acids Research, 10* (1), 61-67 (1982).

17. Dumas, J. P. and J. Ninio, "Efficient Algorithms for Folding and Comparing Nucleic Acid Sequences," *Nucleic Acids Research, 10* (1), 197-206 (1982).

18. Felenstein, J., S. Sawyer, and R. Kochin, "An Efficient Method for Matching Nucleic Acid Sequences," *Nucleic Acids Research, 10* (1), 133-139 (1982).

19. Fickett, J. W., "Recognition of Protein Coding Regions in DNA Sequences," *Nucleic Acids Research, 10* (17), 5303-5318 (1982).

20. Fickett, J., W. Goad, and M. Kanehisa, "A Database and Analysis System for Nucleic Acid Sequences," Los Alamos Sequence Library, LA-9274-MS (1982).

21. Fitch, W. M. and T. F. Smith, "Optimal Sequence Alignments," *Proc. Natl. Acad. Sci., 80,* 1382-1386 (1983).

22. Fox, J. L., "Computer Graphics Aid Study of Molecules," *C&EN,* 27-29 (July 21, 1980).

23. Friedland, P., L. Kedes, D. Brutlag, Y. Iwasaki, and R. Bach, "GENESIS, A Knowledge-Based Genetic Engineering Simulation System for Representation of Genetic Data and Experiment Planning," *Nucleic Acids Research, 10* (1), 323-340 (1982).

24. Gaffney, P. T. and G. Craven, "Use of Computerized Multidimensional Scaling to Compare Immunoelectron Microscopy Data with Protein Near-Neighbor Information: Application to the 30S Ribosome from Escherichia Coli," *Proc. Natl. Acad. Sci., 75,* 3128-3132 (1978).

25. Gingeras, T. R., P. Rice, and P. J. Roberts, "A Semi-Automated Method for the Reading of Nucleic Acid Sequencing Gels," *Nucleic Acids Research, 10* (1), 103-114 (1982).

26. Gingeras, T. R., J. P. Milazzo, D. Sciaky, and R. J. Roberts, "Computer Programs for the Assembly of DNA Sequences," *Nucleic Acids Research, 7* (2), 529-545 (1979).

27. Gingerase, T. R. and R. J. Roberts, "Steps Toward Computer Analysis of Nucleotide Sequences," *Science, 209,* 1322-1328 (1980).

28. Go, N. and H. Taketomi, "Respective Roles of Short- and Long-Range Interactions in Protein Folding," *Proc. Natl. Acad. Sci., 75* (2), 559-563 (1978).

29. Goad, W. B. and M. I. Kanehisa, "Pattern Recognition in Nucleic Acid Sequences. I., A General Method for Finding Local Homologies and Symmetries," *Nucleic Acids Research, 10* (1), 247-263 (1982).

30. Goel, N. S., "On the Computation of the Tertiary Structure of Globular Proteins II," *J. Theor. Biol., 77,* 253-305 (1979).

31. Graff, M., H. Short, and J. Keene, "Gene-Splicing Methods Move From Lab to Plant," *Chemical Engineering,* 22-27 (June 13, 1983).

32. Gunsteren, W. F. van, J. H. C. Berendsen, J. Hermans, W. G. J. Hol, and J. P. M. Postma, "Computer Simulation of the Dynamics of Hydrated Protein Crystals and Its Comparison With X-Ray Data," *Proc. Natl. Acad. Sci., 80,* 4315-4319 (1983).

33. Hackert, M. L., R. M. Oliver, and L. J. Reed, "A Computer Model Analysis of the Active-Site Coupling Mechanism in the Pyruvate Dehydrogenase Multienzyme Complex of Escherichia Coli," *Proc. Natl. Acad. Sci.,* 80, 2907-2911 (1983).

34. Hagler, A. T. and B. Honig, "On the Formation of Protein Tertiary Structure on a Computer," *Proc. Natl. Acad. Sci.,* 75 (2), 554-558 (1978).

35. Harr, R., P. Hagblom, and P. Gustafsson, "Two-Dimensional Graphic Analysis of DNA Sequence Homologies," *Nucleic Acids Research, 10* (1), 365-374 (1982).

36. Howell, J. A., T. F. Smith, and M. S. Waterman, "Computation of Generating Functions for Biological Molecules," *SIAM J. Appl. Math, 39* (1), 119-133 (1980).

37. Howell, J. A., T. F. Smith, and M. S. Waterman, "Computation of Generating Functions for Biological Molecules," *SIAM J. Appl. Math, 38* (1), 119-132 (1980).

38. Isono, K., "Computer Programs to Analyze DNA and Amino Acid Sequence Data," *Nucleic Acids Research, 10* (1), 85-89 (1982).

39. Jaenicke, R., "Folding and Association of Proteins," *Biophys. Struct. Mech., 8,* 231-256 (1982).

40. Jagadeeswaran, P. and P. M. McGuire, Jr., "Interactive Computer Programs in Sequence Data Analysis," *Nucleic Acids Research, 10* (1), 433-447 (1982).

41. Johnson, C. K., "OR TEP-II: A Fortran Thermal-Ellipsoid Plot Program for Crystal Structure Illustrations," *Oak Ridge National Laboratory,* 5138 (March 1976).

42. Jungck, J. R., D. Gregg, and A. G. Dick, "Computer-Assisted Sequencing, Interval Graphs, and Molecular Evolution," *BioSystems, 15,* 259-273 (1981).

43. Kanehisa, M. I., "Los Alamos Sequence Analysis Package for Nucleic Acids and Proteins," *Nucleic Acids Research, 10* (1), 183-196 (1982).

44. Kanehisa, M. I. and W. B. Goad, "Pattern Recognition in Nucleic Acid Sequences. II. An Efficient Method for Finding Locally Stable Secondary Structures," *Nucleic Acids Research, 10* (1), 265-278 (1982).

45. Kano, F. and N. Go, "Dynamics of Folding and Unfolding Transition in a Globular Protein Studied by Time Correlation Functions from Computer Simulation," *Biopolymers, 21,* 565-581 (1982).

46. Kroger, M. and A. Kroger-Block, "A Flexible New Computer Program for Handling DNA Sequence Data," *Nucleic Acids Research, 10* (1), 229-236 (1982).

47. Kuntz, I. D., "An Approach to the Tertiary Structure of Globular Proteins," *J. Amer. Chem. Soc., 97* (15), 4362-4366 (1975).

48. Larson, R. and J. Messing, "Apple II Software for M14 Shotgun DNA Sequencing," *Nucleic Acids Research, 10* (1), 39-49 (1982).

49. Lautenberger, J. A., "A Program for Reading DNA Sequence Gels Using a Small Computer Equipped with a Graphics Tablet," *Nucleic Acids Research, 10* (1), 27-30 (1982).

50. Lee, J. M., J. F. Pollard, and G. A. Coulman, "Ethanol Fermentation with Cell Recycling: Computer Simulation," *Biotechnology and Bioengineering, 25,* 497-511 (1983).

51. Lesk, A. M. and G. D. Rose, "Folding Units in Globular Proteins," *Proc. Natl. Acad. Sci., 78* (7), 4304-4308 (1981).

52. Lilley, D. M. J., "A Simple Computer Program for Calculating, Modifying and Drawing Circular Restriction Maps," *Nucleic Acids Research, 10* (1), 19-26 (1982).

53. McConkey, E. H., "Molecular Evolution, Intracellular Organization, and the Quinary Structure of Proteins," *Proc. Natl. Acad. Sci., 79,* 3236-3240 (1982).

54. "Computers and the Biologist," *Nature, 290,* 914 (1981).

55. Nemethy, G. and H. A. Scheraga, "A Possible Folding Pathway of Bovine Pancreatic RNase," *Proc. Natl. Acad. Sci., 76* (12), 6050–6054 (1979).

56. Novotny, J., "Matrix Program to Analyze Primary Structure Homology," *Nucleic Acids Research, 10* (1), 127–131 (1982).

57. Nussinov, R. and I. Tinoco, Jr., "Small Changes in Free Energy Assignments for Unpaired bnases do not Affect Predicted Secondary Structures in Single Stranded RNA," *Nucleic Acids Research, 10* (1), 341–349 (1982).

58. Nussinov, R. and I. Tinoco, Jr., "Secondary Structure Model for the Complete Simian Virus 40 Late Precursor mRNA," *Nucleic Acids Research, 10* (1), 351–363 (1982).

59. Nussinov, R. and A. B. Jacobson, "Fast Algorithm for Predicting the Secondary Structure of Single-Stranded RNA," *Proc. Natl. Acad. Sci., 77* (11), 6309–6313 (1980).

60. Nussinov, R., "An Efficient Code Searching for Sequence Homology and DNA Duplication," *J. Theor. Biol., 100,* 319–328 (1983).

61. Orcutt, B. C., D. G. George, J. A. Frederickson, and M. O. Dayhoff, "Nucleic Acid Sequence Database Computer System," *Nucleic Acids Research, 10* (1), 157–173 (1982).

62. Osterburg, G., K. H. Glatting, and R. Sommer, "Computer Programs for the Analysis and the Management of DNA Sequences," *Nucleic Acids Research, 10* (1), 207–216 (1982).

63. Osterburg, G. and R. Sommer, "Computer Support of DNA Sequence Analysis," *Computer Programs in Biomedicine, 13,* 101–109 (1981).

64. Pain, R., "Protein Folding by Numbers," *Nature, 298,* 513–514 (1982).

65. Patarca, R., B. Dorta, and J. L. Ramiraez, "Creation of a Data Base for Sequences of Ribosomal Nucleic Acids and Detection of Conserved Restriction Endonucleases Sites Through Computerized Processing," *Nucleic Acids Research, 10* (1), 175–182 (1982).

66. Pearson, W. R., "Automatic Construction of Restriction Site Maps," *Nucleic Acids Research, 10* (1), 217–227 (1982).

67. Periti, P., "A Bayesian Approach to the Recognition of Discrete Patterns with an Application to a Problem of Protein Molecular Structure," *Boll. Chim. Farm., 113,* 187–218 (1974).

68. Plucknett, D. L., N. J. H. Smith, J. T. Williams, and N. Murthi Anishetty, "Crop Germplasm Conservation and Developing Countries," *Science, 220,* 163–169 (1983).

69. Pottle, C., M. S. Pottle, R. W. Tuttle, R. J. Kinch, and H. A. Scheraga, "Conformational Analysis of Proteins: Algorithms and Data Structures for Array Processing," *Jnl. Computational Chemistry, 1* (1), 46–58 (1980).

70. Ptitsyn, O. B., "Protein Folding: General Physical Model," *Federation of European Biochemical Societies, 131* (2), 197–202 (1981).

71. Pustell, J. and F. C. Kafatos, "A Convenient and Adaptable Package of DNA Sequence Analysis Programs for Microcomputers," *Nucleic Acids Research, 10* (1), 51–59 (1982).

72. Queen, C., M. N. Wegman, and L. J. Korn, "Improvements to a Program for DNA Analysis: A Procedure to Find Homologies Among Many Sequences," *Nucleic Acids Reserach, 10* (1), 449–456 (1982).

73. Rackovsky, S. and H. A. Scheraga, "Influence of Ordered Backbone Structure on

Protein Folding. A Study of Some Simple Models," *Macromolecules, 11* (1), 1-8 (1978).

74. Rapaport, D. C. and H. A. Scheraga, "Evolution and Stability of Polypeptide Chain Conformation: A Simulation Study," *Macromolecules, 14,* 1238-1246 (1981).

75. Rodier, F., J. Gabarro-Arpa, R. Ehrlich, and C. Reiss, "Key for Protein Coding Sequence Identification: Computer Analysis of Codon Strategy," *Nucleic Acids Research, 10* (1), 391-402 (1982).

76. Rosen, R., "Protein Folding: A Prototype for Control of Complex Systems," *Int. J. Systems Sci., 11* (5), 527-540 (1980).

77. Rossman, M. G. and P. Argos, "Protein Folding," *Ann. Rev. Biochem., 50,* 497-532 (1981).

78. Sankoff, D., R. J. Cedergren, and W. McKay, "A Strategy for Sequence Phylogeny Research," *Nucleic Acids Research, 10* (1), 421-431 (1982).

79. Scheraga, H. A., "Recent Progress in the Theoretical Treatment of Protein Folding," *Biopolymers, 22,* 1-14 (1983).

80. Scherer, G. E. F., M. D. Walkinshaw, and S. Arnott, "A Computer Aided Oligonucleotide Analysis Provides a Model Sequence for RNA Polymerase-Promoter Recognition in E. Coli," *Nucleic Acids Research, 5* (10), 3759-3773 (1978).

81. Schneider, T. D., G. D. Stormo, J. S. Haemer, and L. Gold, "A Design for Computer Nucleic-Acid-Sequence Storage, Retrieval, and Manipulation," *Nucleic Acids Research, 10* (9), 3013-3024 (1982).

82. Schroeder, J. L. and F. R. Blattner, "Formal Description of a DNA Oriented Computer Language," *Nucleic Acids Research, 10* (1), 69-84 (1982).

83. Sege, R. D. and B. E. H. Saxberg, "A Statistical Test for Comparing Several Nucleotide Sequences," *Nucleic Acids Research, 10* (1), 375-389 (1982).

84. Shapiro, M. B., "An Algorithm for Reconstructing Protein and RNA Sequences," *Jnl. Assoc. for Computing Machinery, 14* (4), 720-731 (1967).

85. Shepherd, J. C. W., "Method to Determine the Reading Frame of a Protein from the Purine/Pyrimidine Genome Sequence and Its Possible Evolutionary Justification," *Proc. Natl. Acad. Sci., 78* (3), 1596-1600 (1981).

86. Shone, J., "Determining the Primary Structure of an Oligopeptide—A Computer Simulation," *Jnl. of Biological Education, 13* (2), 123-126 (1979).

87. Simon, I., G. Nemethy, and H. A. Scheraga, "Conformational Energy Calculations of the Effects of Sequence Variations on the Conformations of Two Tetrapeptides," *Tetrapeptides, 11* (4), 797-804 (1978).

88. Singhal, R. P., R. C. Ray, and L. Dobbs, "Computer Program for Storage and Retrieval of the Nucleic Acid Structures," *Computer Programs in Biomedicine, 14,* 277-282 (1982).

89. Smith, T. F. and C. Burks, "Searching for Sequence Similarities," *Nature, 301,* 30 (January 1983).

90. Staden, R. and A. D. McLachlan, "Codon Preference and Its Use in Identifying Protein Coding Regions in Long DNA Sequences," *Nucleic Acids Research, 10* (1), 141-156 (1982).

91. Staden, R., "A Strategy of DNA Sequencing Employing Computer Programs," *Nucleic Acids Research, 6* (7), 2601-2610 (1979).

92. Stockwell, P. A., "A Large Database DNA Sequence Handling Program with Generalized Searching Specifications," *Nucleic Acids Research, 10* (1), 115–125 (1982).

93. Sternberg, M. and J. M. Thornton, "Prediction of Protein Structure from Amino Acid Sequence," *Nature, 271,* 15–20 (1978).

94. Tanaka, S. and H. A. Scheraga, "Model of Protein Folding: Including of Short-, Medium-, and Long-Range Interactions," *Proc. Nat. Acad. Sci., 72* (10), 3802–3806 (1975).

95. Tanaka, S. and H. A. Scheraga, "Hypothesis About the Mechanism of Protein Folding," *Macromolecules, 10* (2), 291–304 (1977).

96. Taylor, W. R. and J. M. Thornton, "Prediction of Super-Secondary Structure in Proteins," *Nature, 301,* 540–542 (1983).

97. Tolstoshev, C. M. and R. W. Blakesley, "RSITE: A Computer Program to Predict the Recognition Sequence of a Restriction Enzyme," *Nucleic Acids Research, 10* (1), 1–17 (1982).

98. Tometsko, A. M., "Computer Approaches to Protein Structure III. Transformation of Atomic Coordinates," *Computers and Biomedical Research, 4,* 407–416 (1971).

99. Vilenkin, A. and L. Verkh, "Statistical Analysis of DNA Sequences. II.," *Biopolymers, 21,* 1691–1693 (1982).

100. Wako, H. and H. A. Scheraga, "Visualization of the Nature of Protein Folding by a Study of a Distance Constraint Approach in Two-Dimensional Models," *Biopolymers, 21,* 611–632 (1982).

101. Wilbur, W. J. and D. J. Lipman, "Rapid Similarity Searches of Nucleic Acid and Protein Data Banks," *Proc. Natl. Acad. Sci., 80,* 726–730 (1983).

102. Ycas, M., "On the Computation of the Tertiary Structure of Globular Proteins," *J. Theor. Biol., 72,* 443–457 (1978).

INDEX

243